I0094884

The Hospice Heritage: Celebrating Our Future

The Hospice Heritage: Celebrating Our Future has been co-published simultaneously as *The Hospice Journal*, Volume 14, Numbers 3/4 1999.

The Hospice Heritage: Celebrating Our Future

Inge B. Corless, RN, PhD, FAAN
Zelda Foster, MSW
Editors

The Hospice Heritage: Celebrating Our Future has been co-published simultaneously as *The Hospice Journal*, Volume 14, Numbers 3/4 1999.

Routledge
Taylor & Francis Group

LONDON AND NEW YORK

The Hospice Heritage: Celebrating Our Future has been co-published simultaneously as *The Hospice Journal*, Volume 14, Numbers 3/4 1999.

First published 1999 by Haworth Press, Inc.

2 Park Square, Milton Park, Abingdon, Oxfordshire OX14 4RN
52 Vanderbilt Avenue, New York, NY 10017

Routledge is an imprint of the Taylor & Francis Group, an informa business

ISBN 978-0-7890-0847-3 (pbk)

Cover design by Thomas J. Mayshock Jr.

Library of Congress Cataloging-in-Publication Data

The hospice heritage: celebrating our future/Inge B. Corless, Zelda Foster, editors.
   p. cm.
   "Has been co-published simultaneously as The hospice journal, volume 14, numbers 3/4 1999."
   Includes bibliographical references and index.
   ISBN 0-7890-0837-8 (alk. paper)–ISBN 0-7890-0847-5 (alk. paper)
   1. Hospice care. I. Corless, Inge B. II. Foster, Zelda.
R726.8 .H67125 1999
362.1'756–dc21

                      99-049079

The Hospice Heritage: Celebrating Our Future

CONTENTS

About the Contributors   xvii

Preface   xix
Inge B. Corless
Zelda Foster

FOUNDATIONS

Origins: International Perspectives, Then and Now   1
Dame Cicely Saunders

Origins: An American Perspective   9
Zelda Foster
Inge B. Corless

History of the National Hospice Organization   15
Larry Beresford
Stephen R. Connor

ISSUES

Symptom Control in Hospice–State of the Art   33
J. Cameron Muir
Lisa M. Krammer
Jacqueline R. Cameron
Charles F. von Gunten

Spirituality   63
Emily Chandler

Access to Care   75
    Constance M. Dahlin

End of Life Care and Decision Making: How Far
    We Have Come, How Far We Have to Go   85
    Connie Zuckerman
    David Wollner

CURRENT EFFORTS

End-of-Life Care: Challenges and Opportunities
    for Health Care Professionals   109
    Deborah Witt Sherman

Hospice vs. Palliative Care   123
    Patrice O'Connor

The NHO *Medical Guidelines for Non-Cancer Disease*
    and Local Medical Review Policy: Hospice Access
    for Patients with Disease Other Than Cancer   139
    Brad Stuart

Hospice Care and Palliative Care: A Perspective
    from Experience   155
    Paul R. Brenner

Putting Patient and Family Voice Back into Measuring Quality
    of Care for the Dying   167
    Joan M. Teno

Documenting the Impact of Hospice   177
    Melanie P. Merriman

New Initiatives Transforming Hospice Care   193
    Stephen R. Connor

REFLECTIONS AND REMINISCENCES

Reflections on Death in America   205
    George Soros

Personal Reflections   217
    Claire B. Tehan

Reflections on the History of Occupational Stress
    in Hospice/Palliative Care   229
    Mary L. S. Vachon

Hospice Reminiscences and Reflections–An 18 Year Personal
    and Professional Love Affair   247
    Ann MacGregor

The Moment of Death: Is Hospice Making a Difference?   253
    Robert Kastenbaum

Index   271

ABOUT THE EDITORS

Inge B. Corless, RN, PhD, FAAN, is a graduate of the Bellevue Schools of Nursing in New York City, attended Hunter College and graduated from Boston University with a bachelor's degree in nursing, the University of Rhode Island with a master's degree in sociology, and Brown University with a PhD in medical sociology. As a Robert Wood Johnson Clinical Scholar, Dr. Corless did postdoctoral study at the University of California-San Francisco. Dr. Corless served as Program Director of St. Peter's Hospice in Albany, New York, and as a short term consultant for WHO at the Western Pacific Regional Office in Manila. Dr. Corless is the Director of the HIV/AIDS Specialization at the MGH Institute of Health Professions at the Massachusetts General Hospital where she holds the rank of Professor. She is currently working with colleagues in Physical Therapy and Social Work to develop an interdisciplinary Palliative Care Specialization. A Fellow of the American Academy of Nursing and member of the Research Committee of the National Hospice Organization, Dr. Corless has written on hospice, multiple loss, spirituality and on HIV/AIDS. She is the co-editor with Mary Pittman-Lindeman of *AIDS: Principles, Practices and Politics* and with Mary Pittman and Barbara Germino of *Dying, Death and Bereavement: Theoretical Perspectives and Other Ways of Knowing*; and a *Challenge for Living: Dying Death and Bereavement*.

Zelda Foster, MSW, is the former director of a large social work department in a Veterans Affairs Medical Center. She is a co-founder and first president of the New York State Hospice Association. As a young social worker in 1965, she wrote what was considered a seminal article dealing with the conspiracy of silence facing dying patients. She continued and was further propelled into a commitment to improving the care of the dying and the role of health professionals in challenging and impacting the quality of patient care. She has developed homeless, hospital base homecare, employee assistance and adult day programs.

Zelda Foster is a graduate of Brooklyn College and the Columbia University School of Social Work. She has extensively written on psychosocial issues and held graduate school faculty positions. She currently consults on psychosocial programs and end of life care. She is a fellow of The New York Academy of Medicine, participates in The American Red Cross disaster mental health services and is working on a Soros Foundation grant proposal. Her involvement as guest co-editor of the special anniversary edition of *The Hospice Journal* has been rewarding and enriching.

About the Contributors

Larry Beresford, Communications Manager, National Hospice Organization, Editor NHO Newsline and Hospice Manager's Monograph, and author, "The Hospice Handbook" (Boston: Little, Brown & Co, 1993).

Paul R. Brenner, MDiv, Executive Director, Jacob Perlow Hospice, Department of Pain Medicine and Palliative Care, Beth Israel Medical Center, New York, NY.

Jacqueline R. Cameron, MD, MA, Attending Physician, Hospice and Palliative Care, Northwestern Memorial Hospital, Chicago, IL.

Emily Chandler, RNCS, PhD, Assistant Professor, MGH Institute of Health Professions at the Massachusetts General Hospital, Boston, MA.

Stephen R. Connor, PhD, Vice President and Director of Research and Professional Development, National Hospice Organization, Arlington, VA.

Inge B. Corless, RN, PhD, FAAN, Professor and Director of the HIV/AIDS Specialization MGH Institute of Health Professions at the Massachusetts General Hospital, Boston, MA.

Constance Dahlin, MSN, RNCS, CRNH, Advanced Practice Nurse, Palliative Care Service, Massachusetts General Hospital, Boston, MA.

Zelda Foster, MSW, Former Chief Social Work Services, Brooklyn Department of Veteran Affairs Medical Center, Brooklyn, NY; Social Work Consultant.

Robert Kastenbaum, PhD, Professor, Department of Communication, College of Public Programs, Arizona State University, Tempe, AZ.

Lisa M. Krammer, RN, MSN, ANP, AOCN, Nurse Practitioner, Palliative Care and Home Hospice Program, Northwestern Memorial Hospital, Chicago, IL.

Ann MacGregor, Executive Director, Hospice of North Iowa, Mason City, IO.

Melanie P. Merriman, PhD, MBA, Touchstone Consulting, North Bay Village, FL.

J. Cameron Muir, MD, Fellow in Medical Oncology and Palliative Medicine, Northwestern University Medical School, Chicago, IL.

Patrice O'Connor, RN, MA, CNA, Palliative Care Consultant, Board Member; International Work Group on Death, Dying and Bereavement, Board Member; United Hospital Fund of New York, Palliative Care Initiative.

Dame Cicely Saunders, OM, DBE, FRCP, Founder and Past Medical Director, St. Christopher Hospice, Sydenham, England.

Deborah Witt Sherman, PhD, RN, ANP, CS, Assistant Professor and Program Coordinator of the Advanced Practice Palliative Care Masters Program, New York University; and Project on Death in America Faculty Scholar.

George Soros, Chairman, Open Society Institute.

Brad Stuart, MD, Medical Director, VNA and Hospice of Northern California, Santa Rosa, CA.

Claire B. Tehan, MA, Vice President, Trinity Care Hospice, Torrance, CA.

Joan M. Teno, MD, MS, Associate Professor of Community Health, Brown University School of Medicine, Providence, RI.

Mary L. S. Vachon, RN, PhD, Consultant, Psychosocial Oncology and Palliative Care, Sunnybrook and Women's College Health Sciences Center; Associate Professor, Department of Psychiatry and Public Health Sciences, University of Toronto, Toronto, Canada.

Charles F. von Gunten, MD, PhD, Assistant Professor, Medical Oncology and Palliative Medicine, Northwestern University Medical School, Chicago, IL.

David Wollner, MD, Attending Physician, Department of Pain Medicine and Palliative Care, Beth Israel Medical Center; Assistant Professor of Medicine, Albert Einstein College of Medicine, Bronx, NY.

Connie Zuckerman, JD, Associate Director, Center for Ethics in Medicine, Beth Israel Medical Center, New York, NY.

Preface

With this volume, we celebrate the 20th anniversary of The National Hospice Organization and the 25th anniversary of the first hospices in the United States. Hospice Inc.'s home care program, inspired by Florence Wald and other dedicated leaders in New Haven and The St. Luke's Hospice Consultation Team, who were inspired by the late Reverend Carleton Sweetser, each began operation in 1974. The Hospice of Marin was in the process of development as were others that were the initial pioneering programs. This volume is dedicated to and pays tribute to the National Hospice Organization and to the pioneers and founders of hospices in the United States and all who share a vital and enduring investment in hospice care.

The contributors to this volume tell the story of hospice in America not only historically but as an up-to-the-moment state of the art presentation of hospice and palliative care. As we, the editors, of this double edition read each article, we were reminded of our own role in this history. One of us (Zelda Foster) remembers Florence Wald's momentous calling together at Yale in 1966 of leaders and "kindred souls." Zelda had written an article in 1965 in the journal *Social Work* entitled "How Social Work Can Influence Hospital Management of Fatal Illness" This article had come to the attention of Cicely Saunders who asked Dean Wald to invite the author to the gathering in New Haven. The realization that her quest to respond differently to the needs of dying people was a shared mission with others was a monumental moment in Zelda's life. She was privileged to develop a lasting friendship with Florence Wald, Cicely Saunders and later Carleton Sweetser. Ms. Foster watched the birth of Hospice Inc. (now the

[Haworth co-indexing entry note]: "Preface." Corless, Inge B., and Zelda Foster. Co-published simultaneously in *The Hospice Journal* (The Haworth Press, Inc.) Vol. 14, No. 3/4, 1999, pp. xxv-xxvii; and: *The Hospice Heritage: Celebrating Our Future* (ed: Inge B. Corless and Zelda Foster) The Haworth Press, Inc., 1999, pp. xix-xxi. Single or multiple copies of this article are available for a fee from The Haworth Document Delivery Service [1-800-342-9678, 9:00 a.m. - 5:00 p.m. (EST). E-mail address: getinfo@haworthpressinc.com].

Connecticut Hospice) and joined Florence and Henry Wald in writing several articles on the history of hospice. She remembers too the founding of the New York State Hospice Association (NYSHA) and how the founders and early members literally passed the cup around to pay for postage for the Association. What a struggle it was to keep united the "haves and have-nots" (those who were identified as New York State hospice demonstration programs and those who were not). How was it possible to hold a full time position as the director of a large social work department in a veteran's hospital, raise two small children, simultaneously hold three offices in the fledgling New York State Hospice Association and drive periodically to Albany to Board meetings in what always seemed to be an ice storm? Ms. Foster later went on to develop for the Veteran's Administration hospice, home-care, adult day health care, employee assistance and homeless programs.

The editors' paths crossed when Inge Corless moved to New York. Her earlier work in Michigan and developments there became the foundation for NYSHA's charter. Inge Corless had come to New York to assume the role of program director of St. Peter's Hospice in Albany and subsequently was elected to the Board of Directors of NYSHA. In the early 1980s, she chaired the Research committee of NHO. She was awarded a Robert Wood Johnson post-doctoral fellowship to the University of California at San Francisco where her interest in mind/body interaction and the use of complementary therapies and life defining illness were explored. This led to an opportunity to work with individuals infected with the human immunodeficiency virus (HIV) which she did feeling that health care professionals and hospice had a role to play with these individuals. It was a time when some professionals refused to provide care. Dr. Corless, together with Dr. Mary Pittman-Lindeman, edited one of the first interdisciplinary books on AIDS believing that it was essential to examine various aspects of this issue. She continued to work in the field of HIV/AIDS and in the fields of death and dying, and is currently a member of the editorial boards of several prominent journals. She also chaired two Work Groups of the International Work Group on Death, Dying and Bereavement that produced The Assumptions and Principles of Persons Infected with the Human Immundeficiency Virus and the Assumptions and Principles of Spiritual Care, and edited *A Challenge for Living: Dying, Death and Bereavement* and a second book, *Dying,*

Death and Bereavement: Theoretical Perspectives and Other Ways of Knowing (with co-editors Barbara Germino and Mary Pittman).

We are grateful to the contributors to this volume who are a very talented group of individuals. We can readily see from their articles that hospice as a movement and a set of principles and values, grows, changes and lives in new forms. There is a profound knowledge base, an expertise and personal contribution as well as commitment and wisdom. There is the concern for the availability of a wide array of services to be offered to more people as they face the end of their lives. The kind of urgency and mission underpinning hospice as a social reform movement needs continued rekindling, as we have not yet achieved all that is needed. The voices of the contributors to this anniversary issue express the past, present and future hopes not only of these individuals but of the numerous others whom they represent. Happy Birthday NHO.

Inge B. Corless
Zelda Foster

FOUNDATIONS

Origins:
International Perspectives,
Then and Now

Dame Cicely Saunders

SUMMARY. It was because a number of people took time to listen to patients and families facing mortal illness that the Hospice Movement has grown world-wide since it began in the 1960s. The addition of new skills in pain and symptom control, the understanding of the problems faced by families and the need for research and teaching has brought the old traditions in care and caring into the present day. It has shown that it can be relevant in many settings and cultures and in countries with widely different resources. *[Article copies available for a fee from The Haworth Document Delivery Service: 1-800-342-9678. E-mail address: getinfo@haworthpressinc.com <Website: http://www.haworthpressinc.com>]*

KEYWORDS. Hospice origins, hospice history, international hospice movement, palliative care, terminal illness, pain and symptom control, death and dying

I am a part of all that I have met.

Tennyson–Ulysses

[Haworth co-indexing entry note]: "Origins: International Perspectives, Then and Now." Saunders, Dame Cicely. Co-published simultaneously in *The Hospice Journal* (The Haworth Press, Inc.) Vol. 14, No. 3/4, 1999, pp. 1-7; and: *The Hospice Heritage: Celebrating Our Future* (ed: Inge B. Corless and Zelda Foster) The Haworth Press, Inc., 1999, pp. 1-7. Single or multiple copies of this article are available for a fee from The Haworth Document Delivery Service [1-800-342-9678, 9:00 a.m. - 5:00 p.m. (EST). E-mail address: getinfo@haworthpressinc.com].

As I trace the origins of the modern hospice movement I am aware that it owes its inception and development to our experience of listening to patients and their families. I would therefore like to re-write the above phrase as follows: "All that I have met are a part of me" and salute all those we remember as both challenge and reward.

Once again I record the words of David Tasma, the young Jewish man from Poland, whose two phrases "I'll be a window in your Home" and "I want what is in your mind and in your heart" impelled me into this work. From them came the call to openness to all future demands and the meeting together of science and relationships. After his quiet death I knew that we also had to create space for the freedom of the spirit and the personal search for meaning of all who would need our welcome and care.

The seven years as a voluntary R.N. in St. Luke's Hospital (originally opened as a Home for the Dying Poor in 1893) and the seven years of clinical care and research as a physician in St. Joseph's Hospice (founded in 1905) gave me the inspiration to interpret these principles and plan St. Christopher's as the first research and teaching Hospice (opened in 1967). It took nineteen years to build the Home round the window!

Looking back I realize how my own Nursing training during World War II (before the introduction of antibiotics and most of the drugs available now) showed me the importance of attention to detail and personal commitment. So often we had nothing but ourselves to give. The experience of spinal surgery also had its impact, but in many ways it was the years as a Medical Social Worker (or Lady Almoner) from 1947-1951 that helped me to see patients as part of a whole family network, best known as individuals in their own home setting. Medical School in 1951-1958 added yet another dimension and it was during those years that many of the drugs, whose use we now take for granted, were introduced. From text books we find that most of our psychotropic drugs, the steroids and NSAIDS were first used generally during that decade.

Experience in St. Joseph's with 1,100 patients whose notes were analysed and the many tape recordings of their comments made in those formative years 1958-1967, together with meetings with many others concerned with this field of need are, I believe, part of us all today. This has led to the sophistication of the *Oxford Textbook of*

Palliative Medicine and the many other texts now available around the world.

Invalided from nursing, I enjoyed my time as a medical social worker and it was then that I met that first patient and responded to what I interpreted as a call to care for people at the end of their lives. Three years later, after experience as a nurse volunteer with dying patients in St. Luke's and the discovery of a few articles by other social workers, I was told by the thoracic surgeon for whom I was working to embark on yet another career. He said "go and read medicine. It's the doctors who desert the dying. There's so much more to be learnt about pain and you'll only be frustrated if you don't do it properly and they won't listen to you."

In 1957, after medical training, those seven years as a volunteer nurse and the beginnings of a literature search, I wrote for my hospital gazette: "Patients always rely on their own hospital. It seems best that they should stay at home as long as possible and then go to a Home for the Dying if and when it becomes necessary. Continuity of treatment by the doctor in charge should somehow be combined with this. One has in mind some form of Home Care with a doctor visiting from the hospital and a Home in close contact with that hospital, all working in co-operation with the family doctor" (Saunders 1958).

This quite prescient ideal is now approached in different ways around the world. After endless networking, many lectures with the stories of patients illustrated with slides and over fifty articles and with capital from grant giving charities and the general public, St. Christopher's opened in 1967. The U.K. Ministry of Health was persuaded to allocate funding for home care, drug studies and evaluation of the need and impact of the Hospice on the local community and hospitals. Dr. Colin Murray Parkes, known world-wide for his pioneering work in research in bereavement, carried out many of these studies from the time the Hospice welcomed its first patients. This evaluation has now been carried out three times during the past 30 years. Pain and symptom control in local hospitals now approaches the Hospice practice in the memories of survivors while they still fail to reach the standard of psychosocial care or continuity of treatment.

Twycross was invited to develop a planned research programme to compare morphine and diamorphine (heroin) in a double blind study. One hundred, forty-nine within-patient crossover observations from a much larger total input showed no clinically observable difference between the two drugs when given orally on a four hourly regime with adjuvant therapy. This was a most important finding. Diamorphine (our drug of choice at St. Joseph's) is not available worldwide and if we had not been able to point out that it was not the individual drug that mattered so much as the way it was used, we could have had little impact on practice beyond our shores.

Home care from St. Christopher's, planned from the beginning, began in 1969 and has escalated, especially over the last five years until at least eight times as many people are at home on any one day as are in the Hospice beds. Many of these come up to the Day Hospice which carries out an imaginative programme singly and in groups. It was soon shown that the system of symptom control and family support was possible in the home setting.

The relationship with workers in the field in the USA began during the years in St. Joseph's and was especially fruitful. A nursing scholarship from my Nightingale School enabled me to plan a tour of the USA in 1963. By that time I had published a number of articles and a chapter in a cancer text book (Saunders 1960). A booklet based on six articles in the *Nursing Times* (Saunders 1960) served as an introduction to Herman Feifel, whose book, *The Meaning of Death*, was published in 1959 as I was writing my first articles. None of his contributors deal with symptom control (Feifel 1959). I met him in Los Angeles and also met Quint and Glaser in San Francisco and several of the clinical pain researchers such as Beecher in Boston and Houde and Rogers in New York. I also visited Calvary Hospital and St. Rose's Home in New York. Everywhere I was encouraged to develop work in this field. A grant from the Ella Lyman Cabot Trust enabled me to extend the tour and return with the typical reaction "Anybody can do anything" that US enthusiasm can engender.

Most important of all was the contact with Florence Wald, then Dean of the Graduate School of Nursing at Yale which led to a six week lectureship in 1966 and a meeting with Elizabeth Kubler Ross, then carrying out her seminal interviews. Many of us have dated the beginning of the Hospice movement to the opening of St. Christopher's in 1967 but as Clark has recently written "even before St. Christopher's had begun operational life, it had already become a source of inspiration, not only to others elsewhere in Britain but also to individuals and groups overseas, particularly in the United States" (Clark 1998).

Shorter contacts in Europe also revealed the yawning gap in research and teaching and began the international contacts of St. Christopher's Hospice Information Service that have developed into a world-wide network of over 80 countries. It has been important to publish research into the widely accepted myths concerning the control of chronic and terminal pain. As Wall has written "The valiant development of palliative care has succeeded in the face of two common myths which were shared in common by patients and doctors. Led by Cicely Saunders and Robert Twycross, the myths were swept aside by precise and convincing observation. One myth was that narcotic medication inevitably replaced the misery of pain with the misery of an insatiable yearning for narcotics. The other myth was that effective repeated doses of narcotics so rapidly escalated that the drugs were only of use for brief emergency periods" (Wall 1997).

The regular giving of oral morphine that I had first seen to be so effective in St. Luke's Hospital and was able to introduce, research and evaluate in St. Joseph's, first reached the general medical literature in 1963 (Saunders 1963). Other people had indeed introduced four hourly oral doses of morphine but almost invariably added "p.r.n." so that patients had to earn their morphine by having pain first. That change alone transformed St. Joseph's from "painful to pain free" as one of the nuns expressed it. Home, family and bereavement care could develop once its effectiveness had been demonstrated.

From the beginning it was recognised that these basic principles had to be interpreted in different settings. First Florence Wald in New Haven began Hospice Home Care without backup beds and then Carleton Sweetser in St. Luke's, New York set up the first Consultant Hospital Support Team, both in 1974. By 1975 Balfour Mount had opened the first Palliative Care Unit in Montreal. All these developments came after sabbatical visits of the pioneers to St. Christopher's and heralded the now world-wide spread. Hospice was finally established as a philosophy of care, not necessarily confined to a dedicated building.

The now worldwide spread of palliative care grew mainly from the Hospice Movement and both titles are used. Many initiatives were inspired by a growing network between countries with international conferences and many individual visits responding to invitations to share the growing body of knowledge. The work of the World Health Organisation, spearheaded by Stjernsward, lately of its Cancer and Palliative Care Unit, has had an important impact on government policies, education and drug availability (Stjernsward 1997). However, much needs to be done if the millions of people currently suffering cancer pain are to be reached by the well researched and published knowledge that already exists. In many countries morphine is not available for home care or, in some, even in hospitals. Reluctance to prescribe much needed drugs for relief is widespread, even in countries where palliative care is well established.

The recognition of palliative medicine as a specialty with a career path for physicians was made in 1987 in the U.K., Australia and New Zealand. There are now a number of professional chairs in these countries, for example, eight in the U.K. closely linked with General Hospitals, Universities and Centres. Once again, these mainly began from voluntary sector initiative. Even more important for the spread of teaching and practice, in my view, are the 354 hospital teams in the U.K. Here, as in a number of other countries, this seems to be an important way of demonstrating good practice on a consulting basis.

Hospice and palliative care are recognisably based on common principles whether they are being carried out in shacks in Bangalore or huts in Zimbabwe, or hospitals as far distant in resources and culture as Argentina and Japan. Twenty-one contributors to Hospice on the International Scene (Saunders and Kastenbaum 1997) show how the challenge has been taken up in widely different settings. The basic ideas are eminently transferable, as Kastenbaum writes in the concluding chapter (Kastenbaum and Wilson 1997). Hospice care has come a long way in a short time.

There is still much to be learned about the "total pain" first observed in St. Joseph's with the physical, psychological, social and spiritual elements making up the whole experience that needs to be approached if the patient and family are to realise the potential that may be achieved at the end of life. It is their successes to which we should be looking. This sketch of the beginnings of a skilled return to the old values of care and caring shows how much modern medicine had to rediscover. These were not new ideas; the word "hospice" as a welcome to travellers and the sick was first used in Rome in the late 4th Century of the Common Era and taken to denote care for dying people in 1842 by Mme. Jeanne Garnier in Lyon, France. Down the centuries, innumerable unknown people have given exemplary care but the match today between "mind and heart" has opened up new possibilities of humanising life as well as death.

REFERENCES

Clark, D. (1998) Originating a movement: Cicely Saunders and the development of St. Christopher's Hospice, 1957-1967. *Mortality* 3(1), 43-61.

Feifel, H. (1959) *The Meaning of Death.* McGraw Hill Book Company Inc.

Kastenbaum, R., Wilson, M. (1997) Hospice Care on the International Scene: today and tomorrow. (ed. Saunders, C., Kastenbaum, R.) *Hospice Care on the International Scene.* Springer Publishing Company.

Saunders, C. (1958). Dying of Cancer. St. *Thomas's Hospital Gazette* 56(2), 37-47.

Saunders, C. (1960). Care of the dying. *Nursing Times* reprint.

Saunders, C. (1960). The management of patients in the terminal stage. In Raven, R.(ed) *Cancer* Vol 6, Butterworth, London pp 403-17.

Saunders, C. (1963). The treatment of intractable pain in terminal cancer. *Proceedings of the Royal Society of Medicine,* 56, 195-97.

Stjensward, J. (1997) The international hospice movement from the perspective of the World Health Organisation: in Saunders, C. and Kastenbaum R.: *Hospice Care on the International Scene.* Springer Publishing Company, pp. 13-20.

Wall, P. (1997). The generation of yet another myth on the use of narcotics. *Pain,* 73, 121-122.

Origins:
An American Perspective

Zelda Foster
Inge B. Corless

SUMMARY. The birth of hospice in the United States was fostered by the work of Florence Wald, former Dean of the Yale School of Nursing. Her activities are emblematic of the dedication of many other hospice volunteers who made hospice a reality in the United States. Nurturer, humanitarian and visionary, we salute Florence Wald and the many others who have contributed to the change in how end-of-life care is rendered in the United States. Congratulations and well done. *[Article copies available for a fee from The Haworth Document Delivery Service: 1-800-342-9678. E-mail address: getinfo@haworthpressinc.com <Website: http://www.haworthpressinc.com>]*

KEYWORDS. Hospice, end-of-life care, hospice history

As we celebrate the anniversary of the first hospices in the United States and the birth of the National Hospice Organization (NHO), our thoughts turn to Florence Wald. No recognition of hospice in the U.S. could be complete without paying tribute to Mrs. Wald. The history of hospice is replete with heroes. We chose to tell of Florence Wald's contribution because it became a model with national impact. We hoped too that her voice might represent the voices of all our founders. In the accolades bestowed on Mrs. Wald, there is the recognition of hospice as a transforming influence in the care of the dying. This

---

[Haworth co-indexing entry note]: "Origins: An American Perspective." Foster, Zelda, and Inge B. Corless. Co-published simultaneously in *The Hospice Journal* (The Haworth Press, Inc.) Vol. 14, No. 3/4, 1999, pp. 9-13; and: *The Hospice Heritage: Celebrating Our Future* (ed: Inge B. Corless and Zelda Foster) The Haworth Press, Inc., 1999, pp. 9-13. Single or multiple copies of this article are available for a fee from The Haworth Document Delivery Service [1-800-342-9678, 9:00 a.m. - 5:00 p.m. (EST). E-mail address: getinfo@haworthpressinc.com].

9

transformation was led by committed people from all walks of life and from all corners of the United States. In Mrs. Wald's own words, "These accolades overwhelmed me. Knowing the scope and breadth of the hospice movement and how many individuals from different disciplines made exceptional essential contributions to it nationally and internationally, being singled out seems a distortion of reality and simplification of a complex creative process."

Part of that process involved Cicely Saunders who lectured at Yale in 1963 when Florence Wald was the Dean of the Yale School of Nursing. They saw each other at least annually either in England or the United States for the next ten years as interest in care for the dying rapidly evolved. Dean Wald invited Dr. Saunders to Yale in 1966 as the Annie W. Goodrich Visiting Professor and convened a conference bringing together Cicely Saunders, Elizabeth Kubler Ross, Colin Murray Parkes, the Reverend Edward Dobihal, Zelda Foster and others. The event was catalytic joining voices and words that would challenge the conventional wisdom of the times. It gave strength and spirit to those there about better ways of meeting the needs of dying patients and their families.

Two years later, Mrs. Wald initiated a two year study of the needs and responses of dying patients at Yale-New Haven Medical Center. Together with Dr. Morris Wessel, Reverend Edward Dobihal, Dr. Ira Goldenberg and others, Mrs. Wald convened an interdisciplinary team which gave care to those who had less than six months of life remaining. In this manner they identified the strengths and weaknesses of the health care system in helping dying patients and their families. It became clear that the medical establishment was encapsuled in a definition of medical science that valued detachment and more technical and invasive approaches to care. The patient as a person in need of healing, capable of making choices, and expressing feelings and wants was not central to this mode of care. The resistance of hospital and medical practice to palliative care and to respond to what patients and families wanted for themselves quickly led to planning a facility specifically for those who needed symptom control and holistic care. Mrs. Wald along with an interdisciplinary board incorporated a not-for-profit institution that began home care hospice in 1974. Henry Wald, Florence's husband, provided the feasibility study that became the underpinning for the projected building, a free standing hospice later named the Connecticut Hospice. With the help of Henry Wald, Virginia A. Henderson and the architect Lo-Yi Chan, a site was selected and a design developed for a creative and restorative free standing hospice environment. Dean Wald was pivotal in applying for state approval, enlisting in every phase a wide spectrum of support and endowing the institution with a value system encompassing hospice principles. Mrs. Wald left Hospice Inc. in 1975 as a result of internal dissention regarding leadership and authority.

Mrs. Wald turned her energy to the International Work Group on Death and Dying (IWG) founded in 1975, where she initiated the first effort to develop Assumptions and Principles of Care for the Terminally Ill. Later in 1982, she helped broaden the concept of spiritual care for the terminally ill. Florence Wald, Balfour Mount, Samuel Klagsbrun and others felt unsettled in how the spiritual component was integrated in hospice care. While the Anglican Foundation of St. Christopher's Hospice was clear and identifiable, the spiritual component of hospice care in the United States was vague. After a long search for financial support, a colloquium was funded by the Arthur Vining Davis Foundation in 1986. This event brought together diverse thinkers united in the search for meaning and communication about spirituality both religious and secular. The proceedings "In Quest of the Spiritual Component of Care for the Terminally Ill" subsequently was published.

Accolades received by Mrs. Wald are worth noting since their content reflects not only the spirit of her influence on hospice development but also of the value placed on hospice. In 1978, her alma mater Mount Holyoke College at the fortieth anniversary of her graduation conferred upon her a Doctor of Humane Letters stating:

... you brought renewed strength and importance to the profession of Nursing and, at a time when you were entitled to rest on your laurels, you created a new health care institution that led a medical profession tied up in its own technology to face the implications of inevitable death and at the same time restored dignity to the dying and compassionate understanding to the bereaved ...

Your pioneering enthusiasm undiminished, you relinquished your deanship to devote your full energies to the development of a new institution dedicated to helping terminally ill patients and their families face dying as "the final stage of growth. That institution, Hospice Inc., has become a model nationally and internationally."

Yale University honored Florence Wald with a Doctor of Medical Science in 1995 and noted:

> *Mother of the Hospice in the U.S., you have given us a new vision of caring. you have taught all of us how to honor life by accepting death. Your quiet revolution has dramatically changed our national approach to death and dying. Rather than aggressive medical measures that may simply prolong pain, those who are dying and those who love them can now choose compassionate care that eases suffering. As a gifted teacher, you have shared your wisdom with generations of nursing students. And you have taught all of us how to honor life by accepting death.*

In 1996 Florence Wald was inaugurated in the American Nurses Association Hall of Fame at its Centennial Celebration, the first living member to be so honored. Further recognition came with her induction in 1998 into the National Women's Hall of Fame in Seneca Falls, New York. The ceremony was entitled "Come Stand Among Great Women."

In her most recent publication "Death and the Quest for Meaning," Dean Wald traces the changes in health care and medical ethics that led to the acceptance of the hospice movement.

> *Hospices grew throughout this nation first as a grassroots healthcare reform effort. Later health care and governmental planners became increasingly convinced of the financial as well as the quality of life benefits. Consumers grew to understand that they had the right to influence the quality of their remaining life. Ethical and philosophical values regarding self-determination, family and staff support, dignity, interdisciplinary team shared responsibility, and freedom from pain all formed a coherent framework dedicated to a changed perception of what patients and families should receive from health care providers.*

Mrs. Wald's passion about nursing and its power to impact the lives of people is ever present. She advocates for the inclusion of pain assessment as the fifth vital sign as part of nursing responsibility. She also urges that nursing and nurses assume responsibility for end of life care and assemble the appropriate interdisciplinary team.

Florence Wald is part of yet another unfolding crusade. As part of a Soros Foundation grant, Mrs. Wald participated in a feasibility study of the Connecticut State Prison System regarding the resources and needs of prisoners who are terminally ill. She and her colleagues propose the initiation of educational opportunities for caregivers in the prison system to advance their understanding of the needs of dying prisoners. These endeavors are part of the National Prison Hospice Association.

Florence Wald, the "mother" of hospice in the United States, provided leadership for a reform movement that was joined by many others. As she looks to the future, Dean Wald dreams of a family centered, community based helping network shaped as a bridge between illness and health with people caring for themselves and each other to sustain health throughout the life cycle. Nurturer, humanitarian, and visionary, we salute Florence Wald and the many others who have contributed to the change in how end-of-life care is rendered in the United States. Congratulations and well done.

Selected Writings–Florence Wald

Craven, J, Wald, F (1975) Hospice Care for Dying Patients. *American Journal of Nursing* 75(10): 1816-22.
International Work Group in Death, Dying and Bereavement (1979) Assumptions and principles underlying standards for terminal care. *Am. J. Nursing.* 79:297-298.
Wald, F, Foster, Z and Wald, H (1980). The Hospice Movement as a Health Care Reform. *Nursing Outlook* 23(3):173-178.
Wald F (Ed.) (1986) *In Quest of the Spiritual Component of Care for the Terminally Ill.* New Haven: Yale University School of Nursing.
Wald, F (1994) Finding A Way to Give Hospice Care, in Corless, Germino and Pittman (Eds.) *Dying, Death and Bereavement Theoretical Perspectives and other Ways of Knowing.* Boston: Jones and Bartlett publishers, 31-47.
Wald, F (1997) The Emergence of Hospice Care in the United States, in Spiro (Ed.) *Facing Death–Where Culture, Religion and Medicine Meet.* New Haven: Yale University Press, 81-89

REFERENCES

Statement of Honorary Degree, Mount Holyoke Commencement, May 21, 1978.
Statement of Honorary Degree, Yale University Commencement, May, 1996.
Wald, F (1997) Hospices Past to the Future. in Strack (Ed.) *Death and the Quest for Meaning (Essays in Honor of Herman Feifel).* North Vale, N.J.: Jason Aronson, Inc.

History
of the National Hospice Organization

Larry Beresford
Stephen R. Connor

SUMMARY. The National Hospice Organization grew out of efforts by the founders of the earliest hospice programs in the United States to protect their emotional investments in hospice care, to advocate for hospice interests in Congress and other public policy forums, to define standards for the fledgling movement, and to provide education on the nuts and bolts of running hospice programs for others who were interested in starting hospices in communities from coast to coast. Unlike the model of St. Christopher's Hospice in England, which began as a free-standing in-patient facility and later added home care services, most U.S. hospices started as home care-based programs, often largely manned by volunteers. Among the crucial issues that have dominated the work of NHO during its first 21 years were passage and maintenance of the Medicare hospice benefit, ideological battles over the hospice philosophy, and efforts to extend hospice care to other populations, such as people with AIDS. *[Article copies available for a fee from The Haworth Document Delivery Service: 1-800-342-9678. E-mail address: getinfo@haworthpressinc.com <Website: http://www.haworthpressinc. com>]*

KEYWORDS. National Hospice Organization, hospice, hospice in the United States, Connecticut Hospice, Medicare hospice benefit, end-of-life care, "Standards of a Hospice Program of Care", AIDS (acquired immune deficiency syndrome)

[Haworth co-indexing entry note]: "History of the National Hospice Organization." Beresford, Larry, and Stephen R. Connor. Co-published simultaneously in *The Hospice Journal* (The Haworth Press, Inc.) Vol. 14, No. 3/4, 1999, pp. 15-31; and: *The Hospice Heritage: Celebrating Our Future* (ed: Inge B. Corless and Zelda Foster) The Haworth Press, Inc., 1999, pp. 15-31. Single or multiple copies of this article are available for a fee from The Haworth Document Delivery Service [1-800-342-9678, 9:00 a.m. - 5:00 p.m. (EST). E-mail address: getinfo@haworthpressinc.com].

FOUNDATION

Britain's Dame Cicely Saunders is lauded worldwide as the founder of the modern hospice movement. Her great achievement was to wed contemporary scientific insights on cancer pain relief, physical and psycho-social symptom management and grief counseling to a centuries old, Medieval monastic religious tradition of service to pilgrims–both those making their way across Europe to the Holy Land and those on an even greater metaphoric journey from this world to the next. For Saunders and her followers, the modern hospice reflected the word's ancient meaning as a place of rest and refreshment for travelers, combining "the skills of a hospital and the hospitality and warmth of a home."

Even before Saunders' vision of skilled and compassionate care for the dying took concrete form with the 1967 opening of St. Christopher's Hospice, a showcase facility in London and the first true modern hospice, she had been encouraging the efforts of the individuals and planning groups whose dedicated labors later bore fruit as the earliest North American hospices. Through her lectures and informal talks in the United States, starting in 1963, Saunders' eminently practical model of care for the dying provided the inspiration for Americans such as Florence Wald, then Dean of the School of Nursing at Yale University, to build their own solutions to the problems of care for the dying. Wald also followed Saunders' model in painstakingly, over many years, assembling the components of the program that was launched in 1974 in New Haven as Hospice Inc., the first U.S. hospice.

The founders of Connecticut Hospice, as it later became known, and then Hospice of Marin, the country's second program, which opened in 1976 across the continent in California, quickly discovered that as they attempted to realize Saunders' vision in the new world, they were inundated with requests for information and for education by would-be hospice founders in other communities coast to coast. It became clear that a national organization was needed to bring shape and stability to this volatile, loosely defined, rapidly growing movement.

The organization that was developed to provide definition, standards, information, training, technical assistance, public relations, policy leadership and advocacy–all aimed at simultaneously promoting the hospice concept and the needs of the terminally ill in America–was the

National Hospice Organization (NHO), which recently celebrated its 20th anniversary. In those 20 years the U.S. hospice industry has grown from a handful of largely volunteer efforts to nearly 3,000 hospice programs serving over a half-million terminally ill patients annually–or one out of every five Americans dying from all causes.

From early growing pains and doctrinaire struggles to define the movement's shape and its soul, NHO has grown to become a permanent fixture on the health care scene, a respected voice in Congress and in government and a staunch advocate for terminally ill patients and their families in the context of a rapidly changing health care system. While hospices and their national organization face a host of new problems and complications, which could not have been imagined 20 years ago, they continue to represent a philosophy of skilled and compassionate care for the dying and a coordinated, interdisciplinary, patient/family-centered program of specialized services which bears a striking resemblance to the vision first articulated by Saunders.

A NATIONAL ORGANIZATION IS NEEDED

The small community of dedicated but isolated individuals who were launching and running America's early hospices gathered for the first time in October of 1975. Some 57 of them, from 17 states, came to Branford, CT, to learn from the originators at Hospice Inc., including its executive director, Dennis Rezendes. "We were getting a lot of folks beginning to come to observe us, and it was taking a lot of our time," Rezendes says. "I conceived of the idea of putting on a conference–a two-day meeting to do the education wholesale."

Sixteen months later a second national gathering, twice as large, was held at Riverside Hospital in Boonton, NJ, where nurse Marilyn Thompson and hospital board chairman (and Time, Inc., executive) Zachary Morfogen had established the first freestanding hospice unit in the United States. A third national symposium was held a few months after that, in May of 1977, at Dominican College in Marin County, with David English, then with the consulting firm Elm Associates and now CEO of Hospice of Northern Virginia, as conference chair. Marin had obtained a grant from the Henry J. Kaiser Family Fund to establish a formal educational program on how to set up a hospice, and thereby bring some uniformity to hospice development, says the hospice's founder, psychiatrist William Lamers, Jr.

Still, there was too much pressure on the programs first out of the gate. "We were very concerned how this new word 'hospice' would be used. In those early days hospice was a very high-risk venture. Our time, our finances, our professional reputations were on the line," Rezendes says. "It also became clear to me that we would not survive unless we were tied in to the health care reimbursement system–and the reimbursement system would not make big changes just for those nice hospice people in New Haven. One idea follows another. Hospice was going to need a national thrust. So in true American tradition, we created an organization."

At the 1977 Boonton symposium, Rezendes tried to interest others in the formation of a national organization. The response was favorable, volunteers were asked to raise their hands and a task force was appointed on the spot, headed by Charlotte Shedd, founder of the hospice in Buffalo, NY. Rezendes and Morfogen hammered out the proposed organization's original statement of purpose. "It was placed on me, as NHO's first chair, and Dennis (who became the fledgling organization's executive secretary) to plot and scheme [the national organization into reality]," Morfogen explains.

The task force's recommendations for NHO were accepted by those assembled for the third national symposium, along with a charter and by-laws and an interim governing board, composed of Rezendes, Morfogen, Shedd, Barbara Hill from Hospice of Marin, Dr. Robert Brown, medical director of Bethesda Hospice in St. Paul, MN, Dr. Daniel Hadlock, medical director of Hospice of Orlando, FL, and Douglas McKell from Long Beach, CA. A fourth hospice symposium was planned for later in 1977 in New Haven, and the new National Hospice Organization was incorporated, with the pro bono assistance of the Washington, DC, law firm Hogan and Hartson. Rezendes and his staff in Connecticut provided administrative support for this national organization, and the interim planning committee selected NHO's first Board of Directors, with chairperson Morfogen and many familiar names, along with some new faces.

Right from the start a serious potential challenge emerged for the fledgling organization, in the person of Victor Zorza, a well-connected and influential journalist with the *Washington Post*. Victor and his wife Rosemary had written a powerful article for the *Post*, "The Death of a Daughter," describing their 25-year-old daughter Jane's experience in an English hospice. They had formed a national group of influential supporters, called "Hospice Action," to boost the concept in America, Morfogen recalls. "I remember Dennis and myself working very hard at a restaurant in Georgetown, trying to persuade Victor to join us. We realized you couldn't be a national organization with only provider members. You needed those bigger names." Hospice Action agreed to merge with NHO, and all of the organization's attention now turned toward planning a national meeting and coming out party for hospice in America.

This meeting would give focus to all of the grassroots hospice organizing and planning and involvement of individuals across the country. Dr. Josefina Magno, medical director of a pilot hospice project at George Washington University, was engaged as program manager to plan this meeting, which would be held October 5 and 6, 1978, at the Shoreham-Americana Hotel in Washington, in conjunction with the fifth national hospice symposium. According to an advance description in NHO's August, 1978, newsletter, "In the course of the two days, all phases of the hospice concept in England, where it was born, and now in the U.S., will be studied and reported by those directly involved." The organizing theme was "The Coming of Age of the Hospice Movement in North America."

And what a meeting it was! Based on previous symposia, an audience of 200 was expected, but a standing-room-only crowd of 1,200 turned up. The array of speakers was impressive, including Senators Edward Kennedy and Robert Dole, Dame Cicely Saunders from England, Sandal Stoddard, author of the then-current best-seller *The Hospice Movement*, Dr. Robert Butler, Director of the National Institute on Aging, and Joseph Califano, U.S. Secretary of Health, Education and Welfare. Califano announced that the government would soon be issuing invitations for a national hospice demonstration project. National news media highlighted this new organization and movement, including the PBS news program *The MacNeil/Lehrer Report*. That meeting has been described by its planners as the real birthdate of hospice care in America, and the catalyst for launching NHO as a lasting presence on the national health care scene.

THE MEDICARE MIRACLE

Since that auspicious debut, perhaps the single most important and far-reaching event in the 20-year history of NHO and its hospice provider members was the 1982 passage of the Medicare hospice benefit. This surprising legislative victory helped to secure the survival and growth of the hospice movement as a professional health care provider industry, but at the same time it solidified a certain philosophy of hospice care, as well as a structure and configuration of services. The Medicare benefit is what people are most likely to picture today when they think of hospice. Its enactment also introduced financial interests and conflicts, which continue to shape the battlefield for the soul of what has grown to be a $2 billion industry.

Enactment of the Medicare hospice benefit has been described by its co-author, former California Congressman Leon Panetta, as "an organizational and political miracle." The only new health entitlement created during President Reagan's benefit-cutting first term, it was a tale of tiny David overcoming the combined Goliaths of organized medicine and health care.

The benefit's roots lie in the HCFA hospice demonstration projects first announced by HEW Secretary Joseph Califano at NHO's 1978 annual meeting. These were awarded the following year to 26 hospices, providing them with flexible government reimbursement in order to test the quality, cost-effectiveness and fiscal implications of hospice care. Meanwhile, in Florida, hospital system administrator Donald Gaetz and Rev. Hugh Westbrook, who had established Hospice Inc., out of a Miami storefront ministry, were tackling that state's health care Goliaths through the passage of the country's first state hospice licensure law.

"That was the beginning of the Medicare benefit," Gaetz explains. "We found we could give ourselves a legal foundation on which to build hospice programs. But we'd obliged ourselves to provide comprehensive care, and discovered we had no way to pay for it." They eventually met Dennis Rezendes, who knew how the political process worked from his experience as administrator of the City of New Haven. Rezendes was "working the Hill like crazy," trying to find a way for his program to survive after its three-year National Cancer Institute demonstration grant was to run out. The three of them started drawing on their political connections in Washington, DC, and began seeking support among NHO members. When NHO's board refused to go along with their proposed legislative initiative, they formed a separate lobbying organization called the National Hospice Education Project (NHEP).

In the 1980 session, Senator Birch Bayh of Indiana, whose wife had died of cancer, introduced a bill to extend federal disability benefits to the terminally ill. But it was deemed too expensive and it did not advance. The following year Panetta announced his intention to introduce a hospice bill, and the three hospice advocates approached him to collaborate. Their next step was to retain legal counsel, Earl "Duke" Collier with the Washington firm Hogan and Hartson, which coincidentally had written NHO's original Articles of Incorporation in 1978.

"Duke helped us get started, and met Leon Panetta with us. But the job began to get a lot bigger," Gaetz says. The growing demands of this political initiative were then assigned to a young associate in the firm, Ann Morgan Vickery, who Gaetz calls a very fast study. "Ann and Hugh and Dennis and I wrote that bill. Ann's technical expertise was in every comma of the legislation."

The hospice bill was introduced in December of 1981, with Panetta, Rep. Bill Gradison of Ohio and Kansas Senator Bob Dole as principal sponsors. Gradison also provided access to staff of the House Ways & Means Committee, to help with the technical drafting of the bill. NHEP, with the financial assistance of Warner Lambert, had already commissioned a study of hospice's cost-effectiveness, and the Congressional Budget Office added an influential report concluding that the bill would reduce hospital use and thus save money.

Eight months later it was attached as an amendment to the Tax Equity and Fiscal Responsibility Act of 1982, and enacted into law. How was this tiny, quixotic enterprise able to prevail? Observes Gaetz, "We were written off early on by the smart money" in Washington, and thus enjoyed a honeymoon period when those who might have been able to block it paid it no attention.

The hospice bill had other things going for it, as well, Rezendes relates. "As we began pushing the bureaucracy, we kept meeting people who'd say, 'This makes so much sense.'" Another key was a strong grass roots informational effort by hospice directors in the districts of key legislators. Plus, Gaetz says, "We were blessed by the nature of our opponents." These included huge trade associations such as the American Medical Association, American Hospital Association and Blue Cross/Blue Shield Association, whose opposition appeared to be based on financial self-interest.

THE BEGINNINGS OF THE MAHONEY ERA

Through the process of drafting and enacting the Medicare benefit, the small, divided NHO had achieved a reputation for political infighting and organizational conflict. NHO had been operated out of Rezendes' office in Connecticut until the start of 1979, when the association management firm Executives Consultants, Inc., in the Washington suburb of Vienna, VA, was retained. However, working with a consulting firm that did not fully understand the intricacies of the hospice philosophy ultimately became untenable for NHO.

The board several times offered the job of NHO executive director to Josefina Magno, MD, who had done such a superb job in planning NHO's landmark first annual meeting in 1978. But her commitments to two hospice programs in the Washington area prevented her from accepting the NHO position until the spring of 1980. She came on staff half-time in May and full-time in September, just in time for the organization's first full-blown financial crisis.

Magno returned to Georgetown in 1982 and several other executives held the hot seat of managing the contentious organization until November of 1984, when John J. Mahoney, executive director of Boulder County Hospice in Colorado, was hired as NHO President. He held that position until the end of 1997, roughly three-fourths of the young organization's history.

The 1984 annual meeting in Hartford, CT, turned out to be less successful financially than NHO had counted on. For board members, fund-raising had never been a high priority. As soon as Mahoney could straighten out NHO's financial statements, he discovered the organization was $75,000 in debt, a figure which grew to $99,000 by the end of his first year. How does a small organization deal with such a crisis?

"You start by saying no," Mahoney recalled in a 1988 interview. "The first year that's practically all I did. I had to let go of some office staff. We ran the organization with only four paid staff for three months." Bernie Bell, who had lost a son to cancer in 1970 and was a volunteer with the American Cancer Society and Hospice Care of Rhode Island, was asked by NHO to reactivate the National Advisory Council, to help with fund-raising and draw upon the resources of influential hospice supporters in politics, the arts, philanthropy and the corporate world. Bell tirelessly called in personal IOUs, made phone calls, sent letters and helped keep the organization afloat through the worst of the 1984-85 financial crisis, until the next, more successful annual meeting in Washington could put it back on track. A new, more realistic, graduated membership dues structure was also put in place.

Mahoney defines his role and contribution to NHO as "exactly what I was brought in for," to manage the organization and its finances, to make sure there was money in the bank. "They felt they had their bases covered in presenting hospice to the world. They were looking for someone to take care of the office." In this way, he believes, NHO was mirroring the industry it represented in moving from charismatic, visionary founders to people who could successfully run hospice programs day in and day out. Eventually, with Mahoney's leadership and attention to detail, NHO was put back on a solid footing, ready to face the emerging issues in the health care environment, which have kept it busy ever since.

WHAT ELSE WAS NHO DOING?

Much of the crucial early work of NHO, in bringing order and cohesion and national focus to a visionary, inchoate movement, was done through its committee structure. The first five committees formed by NHO's Board of Directors were: Standards and Accreditation, Reimbursement and Licensure, Evaluation and Research, Education and Training, and Professional Liaison, with others added soon after.

"One of the hardest and most important things we did was the standards," recalls Charlotte Shedd, who sat on the first NHO board and on the Standards and Accreditation Committee as it hammered out multiple drafts of its seminal document, "Standards of a Hospice Program of Care." The standards were first presented to NHO's membership at the 1978 annual meeting. Shedd explains, "The standards grew out of the body of knowledge we had accumulated. In order for NHO to survive, it had to be refined and put into writing." The committee met weekends, away from its members' jobs and homes. "The painstaking care we went through is reflected by the fact that the original standards haven't changed substantially," in subsequent revisions.

A major effort of NHO's Public Relations and Information Committee, chaired by Ewart V. Thomas, Director of Philanthropic Programs for the Warner-Lambert pharmaceutical company, was the edu-

cational film *Hospice: An Alternative Way to Care for the Dying.*
Produced by Frank Moynihan of Billy Budd Films in New York, this
film included scenes shot at Riverside Hospice in Boonton, NJ, and in
patients' homes. It was made with the goal of raising public "awareness, understanding and acceptance of hospice," and premiered in
Washington, DC, in June of 1979. Thomas and Warner-Lambert were
staunch supporters of NHO in the crucial early years. He edited
NHO's first newsletters and the company's total charitable contributions to NHO and hospice during the organization's early years have
been estimated at over $750,000.

In 1980 the W.K. Kellogg Foundation of Battle Creek, MI, awarded
three major grants to the hospice industry, one to launch a model
hospice program in Battle Creek. A second paid for a study of the state
of the art in the hospice field by the Joint Commission on Accreditation of Hospitals. This study eventually culminated in JCAH's first
hospice accreditation program, which began surveying hospices according to defined standards in 1984. The third Kellogg grant was to
NHO for education, training and publicity for the hospice industry.
Totalling over $600,000, this grant funded technical assistance staff
for the new organization, allowed it to provide a variety of useful
educational resources to its members and brought new credibility to its
efforts.

Other key efforts from NHO's early days included passage of the
First National Hospice Week, in 1982; the first video public service
announcement for hospice, narrated by actor Jack Klugman; and development of Hospice Pak–a low-cost liability package for NHO
member hospices. This NHO-sponsored insurance package and its
broker, Thomas H. O'Hara, Jr., helped preserve many small hospices
through the liability crisis of the 1980s. Eventually it took on a new
form as the NHO Insurance Agency.

COLLEGIALITY AND PHILOSOPHICAL BATTLES

In the early days of the U.S. hospice movement, a spirit of sharing
and collegiality was celebrated by all who were involved. The first
two U.S. hospices, in Connecticut and Marin County, CA, and shortly
after that in Boulder, CO, and Monterey, CA, among others, were
heavily involved in teaching others how to do hospice care.

But even at the beginning there was a basic polarity or conflict between standards and creativity, Rezendes says. In retrospect, the infighting should not have been a surprise. These individuals were trying to revolutionize care of the dying, transform America's medical system and bring miracles of healing to the lives of the terminally ill. They had seen how the encounter with death can dramatically change people. Some of them had the single-mindedness to devote six to eight years of their lives to painstakingly building their own hospice programs. With such dedication, they could have intense emotional reactions to any issues touching on the philosophy of hospice.

After the tremendous success of NHO's 1978 inaugural national meeting in Washington, by the time of the 1979 annual meeting in Cincinnati, "there were high expectations and a lot of discontent," Howard Bell, founder of the Minnesota Coalition for Terminal Care and the hospice program at Abbott-Northwestern Hospital in Minneapolis, recalled in a 1987 interview. "I came on the NHO board in 1982, and I remember we had a board retreat with an outside facilitator–and we burned out the facilitator. He quit in frustration."

EXTENDING ACCESS TO MORE OF THE DYING

America's earliest hospices were founded by highly motivated, committed volunteers. They knew, deep in their bones, from personal or professional experience, how much the hospice approach meant to dying patients and families, and they had strong opinions about how it had to be done. They often spent years planning and organizing, before starting in with service delivery, and they devoted considerable attention to getting just the right culture for their programs from the very start.

Some of the most celebrated and successful early hospices began in relatively affluent suburban communities, serving a patient population that was predominantly white, middle-class, diagnosed with cancer, anxious to get off the treadmill of aggressive treatments, and with an intact family willing and able to participate in the care at home. There is considerable evidence that hospices have mastered this type of care, becoming the only demonstrated, successful model for the entire health care system of how to bring comfort, dignity and meaning to the lives of dying patients.

But what about other terminally ill patients who don't fit this model? Over two million Americans die every year and hospice, the only large-scale program specializing in care for the dying, has never served more than a fraction of them–despite two decades of steady growth. One way to understand the history of hospices in America over the past two decades, and the simultaneous history of the national organization formed to represent them and advocate for the needs of dying patients, is as an effort to extend this highly successful model of care for a certain narrowly defined patient population into a much larger realm for which it was not quite so perfectly matched.

Perhaps the most striking example of hospice's expansion centers around AIDS–the acquired immune deficiency syndrome. Almost from the epidemic's beginnings in the early 1980s, innovative hospice programs in San Francisco, New York, Los Angeles, Boston and elsewhere were trying to adopt hospice philosophy to the needs of a very different population of dying AIDS patients. NHO helped to disseminate these innovations through the work of its AIDS Resource Committee and published monographs.

NHO co-sponsored the April, 1987, North American Conference on Caring for Terminally Ill People with AIDS, held in Ottawa, Canada, committing its prestige and authority as the voice of hospice in the United States to the importance of meeting the challenge of AIDS. Through gestures such as these and policy statements issued since the epidemic's early days, NHO affirmed that it was not just appropriate for American hospices to enroll terminally ill AIDS patients–it was their positive responsibility to do so. NHO also sponsored a series of regional AIDS conferences in 1988, and in 1994 its AIDS Resource Committee convened an "AIDS Summit," bringing together hospice leaders and representatives from AIDS service organizations, to explore how to enhance the relationship and better define the proper role for hospice in the AIDS care continuum.

AIDS challenged traditional hospice notions on many levels; for example, what constitutes the patient's "family," what does spiritual support mean to marginalized patient populations, and how can hospice provide a safe home dying experience for people who don't have safe homes. Some hospices were among the very first health care providers in their communities to tackle the intensive needs of AIDS patients, playing leadership roles in organizing local AIDS care continuums. Others changed their admission policies and even service configurations to better accommodate AIDS patients. Yet many of the factors that differentiated AIDS care from traditional hospice care, crying out for modifications from established hospice approaches, raised the obvious question: If we make these changes for people with AIDS, why not for all of our patients?

More recently, protease inhibitors and other new antiviral HIV treatments–which have achieved seemingly miraculous results with a disease once viewed as an automatic death sentence–have once again turned providers' assumptions upside down and forced hospices to reconsider how they might answer new unmet needs in this area. Some of the early hospice responses to AIDS, including the model residential facilities Hospice at Mission Hill in Boston and Chris Brownlie Hospice in Los Angeles, closed because of the sudden drop in demand for end-of-life AIDS care. NHO continues to explore ways of extending access to more of the dying through its Minority and Non-Cancer Access Task Forces.

OTHER DEVELOPMENTS AND ROLES FOR NHO

One of NHO's key roles in the past dozen years has been to advocate with Congress and the federal health care regulatory structure on what providers needed to be able to more effectively serve dying patients. The hospice industry has enjoyed an enviable history of success in using Congressional action to extend or enhance the Medicare Hospice Benefit and to pay providers more of the actual costs of providing this care. In 1986, when the original Medicare hospice law was scheduled to "sunset," hospices persuaded Congress of the need to make it a permanent part of the Medicare system.

Subsequent enhancements, often as amendments to the annual Congressional budget bill, made hospice an optional benefit under Medicaid (which 41 states and the District of Columbia have chosen to exercise); created a fourth benefit period extending hospice coverage beyond its original 210 days; locked in annual cost-of-living adjustments in Medicare rates; and set a 95 percent floor on nursing home room-and-board payments for nursing home residents whose facility-based care is covered by the government and who simultaneously elect the Medicare or Medicaid hospice benefit.

This latter issue, how best to cover hospice care in the nursing home and minimize its potential for fraud and abuse, has generated some of the most heated controversy within NHO in the past decade. In March of 1990, Mahoney told the Hospice News Service newsletter, "Our fear is that this new benefit might be misused by different provider groups–nursing homes and hospices–to be paid reimbursement without providing high-quality hospice care. . . . I'm not saying the problem will happen in every case. But it's a concern we'd better address." In 1992 NHO sponsored a bill, H.R. 5502, which would have limited to 50 percent the proportion of reimbursed hospice care which could be provided in "institutions," such as nursing homes, as a safeguard against such abuses. Some providers lobbied vigorously against this proposal, and it never went forward.

Later, the potential for abuse of the nursing home benefit became a major target of Operation Restore Trust (ORT), an interagency fraud-and-abuse initiative launched by the federal Office of Inspector General (OIG) in 1995. Attention to abuse issues in health care generally had been growing, but hospice was added to the list of provider groups to be audited because of problems which emerged in 1994 HCFA audits of hospices in Puerto Rico.

The following year, ORT auditors, looking for similar problems on the mainland, began visiting hospices with significant numbers of long-stay patients (more than 210 days). The auditors concluded that many of these patients were admitted without an appropriate terminal diagnosis, and recommended that the government recoup millions of dollars in Medicare reimbursement from the hospices. Through the resulting controversy and media exposure, NHO tried to work collaboratively with OIG and HCFA, but held firm where it believed government auditors were jumping to unsupported conclusions. Late in 1997, OIG issued two additional reports compiling its data on problems in the hospice industry, one focused on the nursing home benefit and the other on hospice admission and marketing practices. The final report from the OIG concluded that hospice care was being delivered essentially as Congress had intended. Oversight by Medicare fiscal intermediaries continues in the form of Focused Medical Review primarily directed at non-cancer admissions.

Throughout Mahoney's tenure with NHO, the organization has placed an emphasis on maintaining collaborative working relationships with the federal government, contributing input to hospice planning by HCFA, the Veterans Administration, the CHAMPUS health program for military employees and families and other government agencies. NHO representatives were invited to participate in a process of negotiated rulemaking to update the regional hospice wage index, used to adjust Medicare reimbursement rates, starting in the fall of 1994. Since this was a zero sum game, balancing relative winners and losers, cooperation was essential to produce an outcome all providers could live with.

NHO staff were contacted by the Clinton Administration in the spring of 1997, just prior to the announcement of an administration trial balloon proposing to eliminate hospice coverage for nursing home residents. Thanks to NHO's input, the Clinton administration agreed to hold off on this plan, and instead to work out solutions collaboratively with the hospice and nursing home industries.

NHO has also been active in providing input to the Joint Commission on Accreditation of Healthcare Organizations, through its first phase of hospice accreditation from 1984 to 1990, and then again in 1994, when the Joint Commission elected to reintroduce hospice accreditation, this time as part of its home care accreditation manual. For some hospices, these new standards failed to recognize the unique aspects of hospice care, but NHO continues to advocate for the hospice perspective, and is represented on JCAHO's home care Professional and Technical Advisory Committee.

NHO has participated in national end-of-life initiatives such as the Robert Wood Johnson Foundation's Last Acts campaign and has contributed to the national dialogue on such controversial end-of-life issues as withdrawing and withholding food and fluids and physician-assisted suicide. NHO's legal counsel filed influential amicus briefs in both the 1990 Nancy Cruzan case and the 1997 assisted suicide cases before the U.S. Supreme Court.

In a policy first affirmed by its membership at its 1990 annual meeting, NHO has argued that legalizing assisted suicide would be unwise, advocating instead for appropriate hospice and palliative care to eliminate the need for euthanasia. NHO joined state hospice organizations in opposing physician-assisted suicide ballot initiatives, successfully in Washington (1991) and California (1992), but unsuccessfully with Oregon's 1994 Ballot Measure 16, which made that state the first to legalize assisted suicide.

Two Gallup polls of public attitudes, commissioned by NHO, have confirmed that while hospice care is not well understood by the public, most people agree with the basic goals and assumptions of hospice and would prefer the opportunity to die comfortably at home, even though they don't know that this is synonymous with hospice. Bridging this cognitive gap will need to be addressed on multiple fronts, including the Hospice Care commemorative postage stamp which was issued in February, 1999.

Perhaps the most emotionally and artistically satisfying attempt to raise public understanding of hospice was launched at the Corcoran Gallery in Washington, DC, in March, 1996. Sponsored by NHO's affiliated National Hospice Foundation, "Hospice: A Photographic Inquiry" presented the work of five prominent fine-arts photographers, who had closely observed and documented real life in hospice settings. Accompanied by a powerful HBO documentary, "Letting Go: A Hospice Journey," and a diverse educational program developed by Learning Design Associates of Columbus, OH, this exhibit will criss-cross the country through the year 2000, appearing at over a dozen major museums.

PROGRESS ON ACCESS,
BUT QUESTIONS FOR THE FUTURE

Through these controversies and advances, experiments and setbacks, the hospice industry in America has continued to grow. Numbers of hospice programs, of NHO provider members and of patients served by hospices annually have all continued to rise, often by 10 percent or more per year. In 1996 an estimated 3,000 U.S. hospices served 450,000 dying patients. Such growth also gives some indication that efforts to reach out to new populations are succeeding.

The proportion of non-cancer patients has grown steadily, to 40 percent in NHO's 1995 hospice census data, with increasing numbers of patients who have end-stage Alzheimer's, renal, lung and heart diseases. According to NHO's most recent data, 98 percent of hospice programs admit patients with non-cancer diagnoses, 97 percent admit people with AIDS and 86 percent admit terminally ill children. Sixty percent of U.S. hospices now admit patients without primary caregivers, and another 27 percent report a willingness to consider such admissions on a case-by-case basis. The proportion of non-white patients has grown in recent years to 17 percent, inching closer to the racial balance of the U.S. population as a whole.

However, the U.S. hospice industry's recent history of growth now runs into a whole new set of challenges and barriers emerging from the growth of managed care, from changes in the health care system and in medical practice, and from mainstream medicine's recent discovery of the needs of dying patients, since the 1995 SUPPORT study. Such challenges as increased competition from other end-of-life providers, managed care-induced belt-tightening, heightened regulatory scrutiny in the wake of ORT and the new national attention to palliative care have made some hospices wonder if the sky is now falling on them.

There have been a number of important changes in NHO recently in an effort to rise to these new challenges. At the end of 1997 a new President was hired. Karen Davie joined the organization from the United Way of America where she served ably as Chief Operating Officer through that organization's tumultuous times. She envisions NHO as serving four major functions: Advocacy, Professional Education, Public Engagement, and Research. The organization is sharpening its focus to develop competency in dealing with these most important strategic services.

In the area of advocacy NHO recently took the lead in opposing legislation that could have made it more difficult for physicians to control pain. The regulatory concerns of hospice providers are also being more vigorously represented in Washington. Improvements in educational products are being made, a more vocal stance on the needs of the dying is being taken in the public arena, and a number of important multi-site research projects on the outcomes of hospice care are being mounted.

Clearly the next few years will have an enormous impact on the future of hospice care in the US and on the NHO which reflects the movement it serves.

ISSUES

Symptom Control in Hospice– State of the Art

J. Cameron Muir
Lisa M. Krammer
Jacqueline R. Cameron
Charles F. von Gunten

SUMMARY. There are a myriad of physical symptoms which can complicate the care of patients with advanced disease. Without knowledge of and attention to these distressing symptoms, the rest of the work of the interdisciplinary hospice team is greatly hampered. In this article, we review the management of ten prevalent symptoms in hospice care and to identify areas of clinical investigation underway and point to future areas ripe for investigation. *[Article copies available for a fee from The Haworth Document Delivery Service: 1-800-342-9678. E-mail address: getinfo@haworthpressinc.com <Website: http://www.haworthpressinc.com>]*

INTRODUCTION

The care of persons with advanced chronic illness is one of the most challenging areas of medicine. Until recently this area has received

---

[Haworth co-indexing entry note]: "Symptom Control in Hospice–State of the Art." Muir, J. Cameron et al. Co-published simultaneously in *The Hospice Journal* (The Haworth Press, Inc.) Vol. 14, No. 3/4, 1999, pp. 33-61; and: *The Hospice Heritage: Celebrating Our Future* (ed: Inge B. Corless and Zelda Foster) The Haworth Press, Inc., 1999, pp. 33-61. Single or multiple copies of this article are available for a fee from The Haworth Document Delivery Service [1-800-342-9678, 9:00 a.m. - 5:00 p.m. (EST). E-mail address: getinfo@haworthpressinc.com].

little attention from the broader health care community. Those working in hospice for more than 20 years have emphasized the importance of symptom control to the care of the whole person through the interdisciplinary team model. It is unfortunate that basic science and clinical trials aimed at improving our abilities to control symptoms have not kept the same pace of growth as the hospice movement itself. As a result, our knowledge and ability to manage the many distressing symptoms of terminal illness has not advanced accordingly.

Fortunately, the situation is changing. Fueled by the growth and sophistication of hospice programs, home health programs, an international focus on improved pain control, the physician-assisted suicide debate and a responsive pharmaceutical industry, there is a growing sense of importance and an increased emphasis on symptom relief for the patient with advanced disease.

In order to mark the 20th Anniversary of the National Hospice Organization, we were asked to evaluate "where we are" and "where we need to go" in symptom control. In this article we have chosen nine prevalent symptoms which are of inescapable importance in the care of patients with advanced disease. We have attempted to define each symptom in the most comprehensive and practical way and to review the "standard of care" for these symptoms. In an effort to be critical of the standard, we have reviewed the current literature with a search of the MEDLINE listings under each topic in the last four years (1994-98), identified areas of clinical investigation underway and point to future areas ripe for investigation. It will be apparent that, while our efforts to palliate are intense and frequently successful, there is room for improvement and more research.

NEUROPATHIC PAIN

It is probably safe to say that the relief of pain has been a focus of human activity for as long as humans have existed. Yet despite millennia of experience and remarkable recent expansion of our understanding of the pathophysiology and treatment of pain, it continues to be a source of tremendous suffering. The management of neuropathic pain in particular remains one of the most vexing problems in palliative medicine.

When patients use words like burning, tingling, electric shock-like to describe their pain, neuropathic pain should be suspected. It may be constant or paroxysmal and lancinating. The clinical findings of allo-dynia, dysesthesia and hyperalgesia appear to be due to abnormally exaggerated pain responses to normally innocuous or mildly irritating stimuli.[1] Although there is much agreement among clinicians about what constitutes "neuropathic" pain, understanding of its precise pa-thophysiology remains surprisingly obscure,[2,3] and much of our prac-tice remains guided only by anecdotal experience.

Pharmacologic interventions are usually guided initially by the clin-ical presentation and proposed mechanism of sensory transmission and central processing. Current agents in use include opioids (though their relative benefit in the treatment of neuropathic pain is hotly contested and will not be addressed here), antidepressants, anticonvul-sants, local anesthetics (oral and parenteral), agents that modify sym-pathetic neurotransmission, and modulators of N-methyl-D-aspartate receptors.

Tricyclic antidepressants such as amitriptyline and desipramine are usually first line therapy for continuous dysesthetic pain (based largely on anecdote and studies of diabetic neuropathy and postherpetic neu-ralgia).[4,5,6] The role of the selective serotonin-reuptake inhibitor class of antidepressants is unclear. Although most studies have shown no benefit, paroxetine, a newer SSRI antidepressant, has been reported to be of benefit.[7] Anticonvulsants such as carbamazepine, valproic acid and phenytoin have proved helpful as first-line therapy for lancinating, paroxysmal pain.[8,9] There is much interest in gabapentin, a newer anticonvulsant which has been reported to be effective for a variety of neuropathic pains.[10,11,12] Baclofen, a central GABA-B agonist, ap-pears to relieve lancinating or paroxysmal pain independent from its role in relieving spasticity.[13,14] Calcitonin also appears to have central analgesic activity and has been reported to be useful in the treatment of sympathetically maintained pain.[15]

A new mechanism for pain-relief seems to be at the level of the sodium channel in its role in propagating pain signals. There has been ongoing interest in the role of sodium channel blocking local anesthet-ics such as lidocaine, mexiletine, and flecainide but reports of efficacy have been mixed.[16,17,18,19] Newer agents (such as SNX-111) are in development.

Some types of neuropathic pain seem to be mediated by complex interactions between spinal alpha-2 receptors and poorly defined en-dogenous systems. This has led to the use of clonidine and other alpha-2 adrenergic agonists for the management of this type of pain, resulting in diminished nociceptive input to central processing centers and decreased sympathetic outflow. In a recent randomized, double-blind trial, Curatolo et al. found that epidural clonidine inhibited temporal summation of afferent impulses which should subsequently diminish spinal hyperactivity and reduce pain.[20] In addition, Eisenach et al. found that epidural clonidine provided significant relief for patients with advanced cancer and severe pain.[21]

The role of N-methyl-D-aspartate (NMDA) receptors in the development of dorsal horn neuronal hyperactivity is currently an area of intense scrutiny. Ketamine, a dissociative anesthetic is also an NMDA receptor antagonist. It has been used in patients with severe pain refractory to very high doses of opioids as well as adjuvant analgesics, resulting in improved pain control and a diminution of opioid doses.[22,23,24] Unfortunately, ketamine can cause psychotomimetic effects and severe dysphoria, necessitating the concomitant use of benzodiazepines. In a search for clinically useful agents without such devastating side effects, methadone, dextromethorphan and dextropropoxyphene have seemed promising.[25,26] Pud et al. recently reported that amantadine, which shows NMDA-receptor antagonist activity, afforded significant relief to cancer patients with severe pain, had a longer duration of action than ketamine, and caused no dysphoria.[27]

Other interventions reported to be helpful include topical preparations of capsaicin and lidocaine, anesthetic and neurosurgical procedures, transcutaneous electrical nerve stimulation (TENS) and acupuncture.

In summary, there are a plethora of poorly investigated agents that appear to be clinically useful at least in some patients. Advances in our ability to manage neuropathic pain requires improved understanding of the mechanisms of sensory transmission in the peripheral and central nervous systems coupled with rigorous testing of existing medications and an ongoing search for novel agents.

DYSPNEA

Dyspnea is a frequent and devastating symptom experienced by many patients with advanced illness. It has been reported to occur in 21%-75% of patients in the days or weeks before death.[28-33] Dyspnea is the *subjective* experience of labored or difficult breathing which, akin to pain, is often challenging to assess. The intensity of dyspnea can be quantified using visual analogue, numerical, and verbal scales,[29] such as the Edmonton Symptom Assessment System[34] and the Support Team Assessment Schedule.[30]

The etiology of dyspnea may be complex and multifactorial (see Figure 1). Many of these etiologies can be effectively treated. For example, antibiotics can be used to treat pneumonia, diuretics to treat congestive heart failure, blood transfusions to treat anemia, and thoracenteses to treat pleural effusions.

The pathophysiology of dyspnea is not fully understood (see Figure 2). Either separately or in combination the stimulation of cortical centers (anxiety or somatization), lung mechanoreceptors (embolism, edema, other) and lung chemoreceptors (abnormal serum gases) can trigger the respiratory center of the medulla to affect both respiratory drive and produce the sensation of breathlessness.[29]

Pharmacological Treatment

The standard approach to managing dyspnea consists of pharmacological therapy with oxygen, opioids, and anxiolytics, while corticosteroids and bronchodilators may be helpful in some patients.

FIGURE 1. Causes of Dyspnea

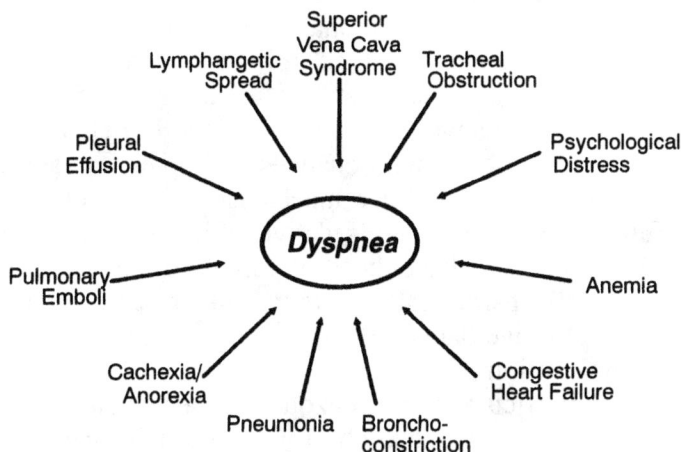

FIGURE 2. Pathophysiology of Dyspnea

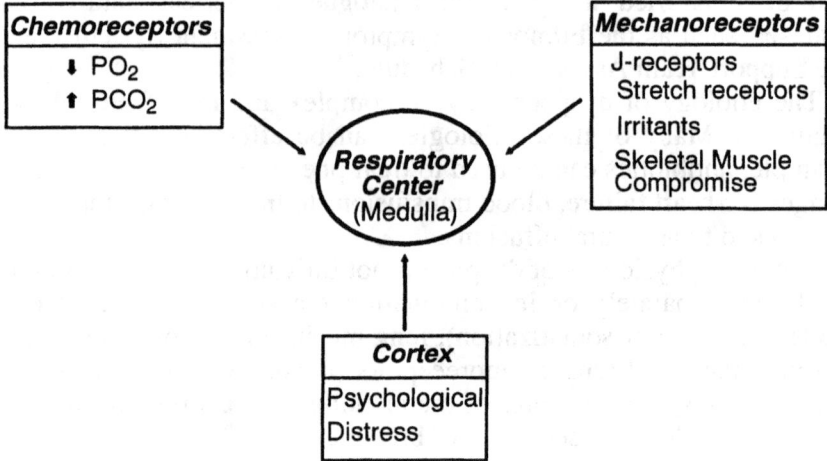

Oxygen therapy is most helpful for patients with documented hypoxemia who report symptomatic benefit from correction of the hypoxemia. A therapeutic trial is suggested. It is important to recognize that there can be a significant placebo effect of supplemental oxygen, thus relief of dyspnea may be due to the connotation of "support," rather than the physiologic effects of the oxygen.

Opioids are the mainstay of pharmacological relief of dyspnea. Although the mechanism by which opioids relieve dyspnea remain unclear, it has been suggested that they act both at peripheral opioid receptors in the lung as well as at central sites. Relief from dyspnea does not seem to correlate with changes in respiratory rate or blood gas concentrations,[37] thus other mechanisms (favorable effects on cardiac function and systemic sedative effects) have been postulated.[28] While opioids have been reported to be effective when administered orally, parenterally, rectally, and via nebulizer, there is no consensus or definitive data on the optimal drug, dose, frequency and route of administration.

Anxiolytics, particularly the benzodiazepines (such as lorazepam) and the phenothiazines (such as chlorpromazine), have been reported to be advantageous when treating dyspnea. Benzodiazepines have been demonstrated to relieve dyspnea and improve exercise tolerance in patients with COPD.[38] It has been suggested that these drug classes are helpful when there is concomitant anxiety, panic or somatization.

Corticosteroids are indicated when an inflammatory process is suspected to underlie dypnea–airway obstruction from COPD or asthma, lymphangitic carcinomatosis, tracheal impingement, and superior vena cava obstruction. Although there is little evidence as to which steroid is preferred for treating respiratory symptoms, dexamethasone (with a long half-life of 36-54 hours permitting once daily dosing, and low mineralocorticoid activity minimizing fluid retention) seems most appropriate.

Bronchodilators (albuterol), given orally or nebulized, are useful for bronchospasm, while the methylxanthines (aminophylline/theophylline), in addition to their bronchodilatory effect, may exert an additional benefit of stimulating the heart and improving respiratory muscle strength.[30]

Several uncontrolled and retrospective chart reviews have been published supporting the use of nebulized morphine.[35] Although attractive in theory, as nebulized morphine has been postulated to exert a beneficial local effect on the airways without systemic side effects, a recent randomized controlled trial demonstrated no difference between nebulized morphine and placebo.[36] Further studies are needed to assess the role of nebulized morphine in dyspnea.

Nonpharmacologic Therapy

Nonpharmacologic interventions are essential adjuvants in palliating dyspnea.[28] When used in conjunction with pharmacological therapies, these measures can impart significant relief of dyspnea for many patients. Chest physiotherapy is helpful in mobilizing and expectorating thick sputum. Just the simple intervention of fresh flowing air, from a window or fan, has been postulated to relieve the sensation of dyspnea through pathways medicated by the trigeminal nerve. Supportive counseling, relaxation techniques, biofeedback, guided imagery, therapeutic touch, aromatherapy, acupuncture, music and art therapy, have all been observed to improve dyspnea. Definitive research to support these observations would provide tremendous support for their use.

CONSTIPATION

Constipation is characterized by the passage of small hard feces infrequently and with great difficulty.[39,40] This highly prevalent symptom exists in approximately 50% of patients admitted to palliative care units.[41] Associated symptoms include abdominal discomfort, flatulence, bloating and a sensation of incomplete evacuation. Unrelieved constipation may lead to anorexia, nausea and vomiting, abdominal distention, overflow diarrhea, urinary hesitation or incontinence, intestinal obstruction, and delirium.

The etiology of constipation in end stage disease is multifactorial (see Table 1).[40-42] The underlying mechanisms of constipation are largely related to alterations in intestinal motility. A history and physical examination is often sufficient to make the diagnosis. However an abdominal radiograph may be needed in some cases.[40]

Laxative therapy remains the mainstay for an effective bowel regimen. The goal of treatment is to produce a comfortable defecation and to relieve associated symtpoms rather than to achieve a specific frequency of evacuation. The choice of laxative depends on the mechanism of action of available agents, the characteristics of the stool, the etiology of constipation and acceptability to the patient. Available laxatives may be classified in the following way.[39]

TABLE 1. Causes of Constipation in Terminally Ill Patients

Associated with Debility	*Specific Pathology*	*Drugs*
Anorexia	Hypercalcemia	Opioids
Inactivity	Hypokalemia	Non-steroidal Anti-inflammatory Agents
Weakness	Spinal Cord Compression	Anticholinergics
Poor Nutrition	Depression	Antiemetics
Confusion	Intra-abdominal Tumor	Antidepressants
Poor Fluid Intake	Pelvic Disease	Neuroleptics
Inadequate Dietary Fiber	Hypothyroidism	Antispasmodics
Inability to Reach Toilet/ Suboptimal Position		Antihypertensive Agents

Predominantly Softening

Oral stool softeners increase fecal bulk and lead to a reflexive stimulation of peristalsis. *Surfactant laxatives* (e.g. docusate sodium), act as detergents to increase water retention and subsequently soften stool. *Osmotic laxatives* (e.g., lactulose) exert an osmotic effect to retain water in the intestinal lumen; larger doses may cause bloating and colic. *Bulk forming agents* (methyl cellulose) soften hard stool and make loose stools firmer; in essence they are stool normalizers. These agents are less useful in terminally ill patients because of the large volume of water needed. *Saline laxatives* (magnesium sulfate) increase the intraluminal volume osmotically. *Lubricant laxatives* (mineral oil) coat the stool surface allowing for easier passage of stool.[39,40]

Predominantly Peristalsis Stimulating

Oral stimulant laxatives (anthracenes–senna, danthron) enhance intestinal fluid secretion which in turn improves fecal consistency. Additionally, they stimulate the myenteric plexus to induce peristalsis as well as increase water retention. The combination of an oral stimulant with stool softeners is highly effective in both the prophylaxis and treatment of opioid-induced constipation.[39,41]

Rectal laxatives are occasionally used if the oral route is contraindicated or has failed. They are available as suppositories (bisacodyl, glycerine) and as enemas (phosphate, arachis oil). Their mechanism of action is similar to the oral agents.

Treatment should be focused on *prevention* of constipation; therefore at the onset of opioid use, laxative therapy should be initiated.

Anecdotal evidence supports the use of gastrointestinal pro-kinetic drugs (e.g., metoclopramide, cisapride) to treat refractory constipation. Future directions include the use of poorly absorbed opiate antagonists (similar to naloxone) to treat opioid-induced constipation.

DIARRHEA

Diarrhea is the discharge of abnormally frequent loose stool. Excluding patients with AIDS, it is a less prevalent symptom than constipation in terminally ill patients. Approximately 10% of patients with advanced disease suffer from diarrhea.[40] Diarrhea can be a debilitating and a dehumanizing condition which can adversely affect personal dignity and quality of life.

A diarrheal assessment includes a comprehensive history, noting stool frequency, quantity, and consistency; and a physical examination to rule out intestinal obstruction and fecal impaction. Intestinal motility strongly influences the absorption/secretion relationship of the bowel. The most common cause of diarrhea in end stage patients is the misuse of laxatives. Malignant obstruction and fecal impaction with overflow incontinence are the second most prevalent etiologies (see Table 2). It is important to recognize that untreated diarrhea may lead to dehydration, fatigue, loss of electrolytes and albumin, weight loss, declining immune function, increased risk of skin ulceration and systemic infection.

Beyond reversing the underlying etiology, the general treatment of diarrhea includes supportive measures such as replenishing fluid if

TABLE 2. Causes of Diarrhea in End Stage Disease

Drugs	Laxatives
	Antibiotics
	Antacids
	Chemotherapy
	NSAIDs
Obstruction	Intestinal
	Fecal Incontinence
Radiation	
Tumor	Colon/Rectal
	Pancreatic
	Pelvic
Infection	
Malabsorption	Gastrectomy
	Ileal Resection
	Colectomy
Diet	Bran
	Fruit
	Alcohol
	Dairy Products
Enteral Feedings	

dehydration is suspected (oral route preferred) and initiating a diet of clear liquids and simple carbohydrates. Persistent diarrhea may require antidiarrheal agents. These agents are classified as absorbent, adsorbent, mucosal prostaglandin inhibitors and opioids. Absorbent agents (methyl cellulose) absorb water to form a colloidal mass. Adsorbent antidiarrheal medications (attapulgite) non-specifically adsorb dissolved substances such as bacteria, toxins, and water. These two categories are only modestly effective for patients with continuous large-volume diarrhea. Mucosal prostaglandin inhibitors (bismuth subsalicylate) reduce water and electrolyte secretion from the intestinal wall. Opioid agents (e.g., loperamide) decrease peristalsis in the colon by way of specific intestinal receptors. The addition of anticholinergic agents (such as atropine) with an opiate (diphenoxylate) may provide additional benefit, but may also cause cramping. Additionally, secretory diarrhea (such as from chemotherapy or HIV) has been successfully treated with octreotide.[39,40] Future research into broader applications of octeotride as well as such novel agents as peptide YY (also thought to reduce intestinal fluid secretion) is needed.

NAUSEA AND VOMITING

Nausea and vomiting are frequent and distressing symptoms. The incidence of nausea in terminally ill patients is approximately 60%, while another 30% experience vomiting.[44-46] The pathophysiology of nausea and vomiting is complex and multifactorial. Figure 3 portrays the neural pathways and associated neurotransmitter receptors which mediate nausea and vomiting. It is important to understand the pathways and receptors involved in the emetogenic process as this permits a more precise approach to diagnosis and treatment.[47-49]

A meticulous history and physical examination will usually suggest an etiology for nausea and vomiting. The goal of treatment is directed at reversing the underlying cause and selecting the appropriate pharmacotherapy. Table 3 lists the common causes of vomiting in terminally ill patients.[47,50]

Emesis due to cortical stimulation may be ameliorated by using corticosteroids (e.g., dexamethasone), anxiolytics (lorazepam) and cannabinoids (tetrahydrocannibinol). Vomiting induced by stimulation of the chemoreceptor trigger zone can be treated with dopamine antagonists (haloperidol, prochlorperazine) antihistamines, anticholergics,

FIGURE 3. Pathophysiology of Nausea and Vomiting with Associated Neuro-transmitter Receptors

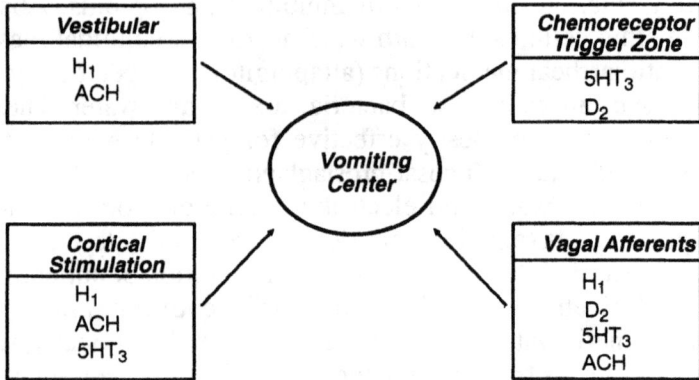

ACH	=	Acetylcholine
D_2	=	Dopamine
H_1	=	Histamine
$5HT_3$	=	Serotonin

and selective serotonin antagonists (ondansetron, granisetron). Nausea and vomiting associated with stimulation of the vestibular apparatus is best treated with such agents as antihistamines and anticholinergics (scopolamine). Emesis associated with vagally mediated peripheral afferents, may be alleviated when using dopamine antagonists, serotonin antagonists, and prokinetic agents (metoclopramide, cisapride).[48,50]

Often, the underlying mechanism may be unclear and/or several different mediators are involved in triggering emesis. Therefore, successful therapy may require combinations of agents directed against each receptor involved rather than using one drug which weakly antagonizes several receptors.[47] Nausea and vomiting can be controlled in over 90% of terminally ill patients.[51]

Non-pharmacologic measures for palliation of nausea and vomiting include supportive therapy, distraction, relaxation, guided imagery, acupuncture/accupressure, and avoidance of unpleasant odors.

Research on antiemetics has been one of the most prolific areas of investigation in recent years. Work is ongoing in attempts to identify new antiemetic agents (e.g., NK1 receptor antagonists, and Substance P inhibitors).

TABLE 3. Common Causes of Vomiting in Terminally Ill Patients

1) Drugs–Opioids, Chemotherapy, Digoxin, Estrogens, Antibiotics, Alcohol
2) Distortion of Gastrointestinal Tract
3) Gastric Etiologies (gastritis, ulceration, gastroparesis, gastric stasis, gastric cancer)
4) Visceral Distention (liver metastases)
5) Raised Intracranial Pressure (tumor, bleeding, metastases, cerebral infection)
6) Metabolic Derangement (renal failure, ketoacidosis, hypercalcemia, infection)
7) Pelvic or Abdominal Radiotherapy
8) Psychological and Emotional Factors (pain, anxiety, fear)

BOWEL OBSTRUCTION

Malignant bowel obstruction (MBO) is a fairly common entity that is particularly challenging to palliate. It is estimated that 3% of all persons with advanced cancers develop malignant bowel obstruction.[52,53] Of these, ovarian (5-42%) and colon (10-28%) carcinomas have the highest likelihood of developing MBO.[53] Many of the cases of malignant bowel obstruction arise in malnourished, debilitated, high-risk patients who have an estimated peri-operative mortality of 12% to 33%.[53] Further, many of these patients are found to be "inoperable" (5% to 50%). For those patients with inoperable MBO, medical management has been employed as the principle means of therapy. Interestingly, the Medline search for intestinal obstruction revealed fifty articles in the past four years, of which 44 related to reports of improved outcome utilizing new metal stents. Only six were related to medical management and are summarized below.

The standard approach to inoperable MBO has been supportive therapy with NG tube, IV fluids, analgesia with an opioid (morphine) with or without co-analgesic adjuvants (NSAIDs, steroids), anti-spasmodics (hyoscine or scopolamine), and anti-emetics (haloperidol, 5HT-3 antagonists). Given the frequency of MBO, it is surprising how scant the data is for these therapies. Generally, patients do not enjoy prolonged NG tube placement–"prolonged conservative treatment using nasogastric suction and intravenous fluids only adds to the discomfort of an already terminally ill patient"[54]–and it is often ineffective in alleviating nausea and vomiting. Baines et al. were the first to describe successful medical management of bowel obstruction without the use of an NG tube, thus their use should be considered a bridging procedure until pharmacological management can be maximized. Most patients with MBO have continuous abdominal pain (92%) and/or intestinal colic (72%-76%). The two pains of MBO are usually treated with the combination of opioids and antispasmodics. Anecdotal case reports have supported the benefits of corticosteroids in MBO, presumably by decreasing the peritumoral edema, but no clinical trials have been performed. Further benefits of the antispasmodic hyoscine were reported by Ventafridda's group who found that it reduced secretions as well as pain in patients with MBO referred to a palliative care service, and that NG tubes were able to be removed with good symptom control until death.[55]

Nausea and vomiting associated with MBO is perhaps the most distressing symptom and challenging to ameliorate. Nearly all patients with MBO have nausea and vomiting (68%-100%). Haloperidol is considered the first line therapy because of its ability to be given safely via a syringe driver,[52] along with the discontinuation of pro-kinetic agents such as metoclopramide and cisapride. The benefits of the 5-HT3 antagonists (ondansetron, granisetron) in obstruction is unclear. While they have been shown to benefit chemotherapy and radiation induced nausea, there are no clinical trials data to support their use in MBO. There are, however, case reports of benefits of 5-HT3 antagonists in MBO, and a study suggesting that patients with MBO from ovarian cancer have higher urine serotonin (5-HT).[56]

There is a growing body of basic science and anecdotal evidence to support the use of octreotide in the management of inoperable MBO to control spasmodic pain to decrease secretions and to decrease nausea and vomiting. Octreotide, which is a synthetic analog of somatostatin with a longer half-life, causes inhibition of gastric acid and pancreatic enzyme secretion. It also inhibits neurotransmission in peripheral nerves of the GI tract leading to decreased peristalsis and a decrease in splanchnic blood flow. There is also some indication that octreotide additionally inhibits the function of activated immune cells and may have a central opioid-like function.[57,58] Thus it has multiple potentially beneficial effects on MBO and is well tolerated. Further research might include combinations of octreotide, steroids, hyoscyamine, 5-HT3 antagonists and determining the appropriate role of metal stents for management of this most distressing syndrome.

ANOREXIA/CACHEXIA SYNDROME

Anorexia (the loss of appetite) and cachexia (involuntary weight loss, weakness, lean body wasting and poor performance status) accompany many advanced diseases.[59] Cachexia is a prevalent (> 80%) and disturbing symptom occurring in most patients with advanced cancer and AIDS, and is the primary cause of death in up to 22% of patients with advanced cancer.[60] Cachexia is also more common in older patients and becomes more prevalent as disease progresses.[61] The diagnosis of cachexia is straightforward, based upon a positive clinical history, the presence of substantial weight loss and the physical examination. Plasma albumin concentration is usually decreased, though its measurement (or that of any other laboratory parameters) is not necessary.[61]

The etiology of anorexia/cachexia is incompletely understood and is likely multifactorial. Three potential mechanisms have been proposed: malabsorption, decreased caloric intake and metabolic abnormalities. Of these, the emerging view is that cachexia is predominantly caused by metabolic abnormalities mostly related to circulating cytokines (TNF, IL-1, IL-6). While decreased caloric intake seems plausible, many studies evaluating the benefits of aggressive total parenteral or enteral nutrition show no improvement in survival. Most published studies did not assess patient symptoms, but anecdotal evidence supports the conclusion that they are not improved. Anorexia is thought to result from the catabolic effects of cytokines; thus anorexia and cachexia are both thought to be secondary to systemic cytokine shower rather than anoraxia directly causing cachexia, as previously thought.

Pharmacological interventions have focused on appetite stimulation. Corticosteroids stimulate appetite and improve weakness without increasing body weight,[62] but their effects are short lived (about 3-4 weeks). Dronabinol, an orally active cannabinoid, improves AIDS-related cachexia, yet it also increases appetite without significant weight gain.[63-65] Furthermore, dronabinol has significant (dysphoric) CNS side effects which appear to be more prevalent in older patients. Cyproheptadine (blocks serotonin-mediated inhibition of appetite), hydrazine sulfate (inhibits gluconeogenesis) and pentoxifylline (inhibits tumor necrosis factor) have been evaluated in randomized trials and have not had a significant impact in patients with cancer cachexia[66-68] Megestrol acetate at high doses is the most potent appetite stimulant available and has been shown to lead to improvement in weight gain with a dose response relationship.[69-71] Interestingly, megestrol did not lead to an increase in lean body mass[72] and this is the outcome measure that is most likely to correlate with strength, endurance, performance status and ultimately prognosis. The anabolic steroids (oxandralone, nandrolone, testosterone, etc.) have been shown to improve lean body mass in patients with AIDS. Human growth hormone has been shown to have similar effects in patients with AIDS as well as the frail elderly. Clearly, further research is needed to understand this syndrome and better treat our patients.

ASTHENIA/FATIGUE

The distinctions between asthenia and fatigue are often blurred by a lack of common language for a set of symptoms that until recently has received little attention in the literature. Asthenia (*Asthenos* from Greek: the absence or loss of strength) is defined as a lack of strength, diminution of vital power, weakness and debility. Originally, asthenia was felt to represent the natural effect of systemic disease on the person–often in the form of a myelopathy.[73] In 1982, Theologides expanded the definition to include the mental and emotional components: "a systemic disability characterized physically by generalized weakness, loss of strength, and easy fatigability of the muscles and mentally by the diminished capacity for intellectual endeavors and an emotional lability or apathy."[74] Others have stated that asthenia represents pathologic levels of fatigue. Bruera and colleagues stated that asthenia is a combination of the symptoms of fatigue and weakness.[75] For simplicity and clarity we are considering them together as set forth in the Oxford text as being defined within the context of three major symptoms:

1. easy tiring and decreased capacity to maintain performance;
2. generalized weakness defined as the anticipatory sensation of difficulty in initiating a certain activity; and

3. mental fatigue defined as the presence of impaired mental concentration, loss of memory, and emotional lability.[84]

Fatigue has been identified as one of the most prevalent and disturbing symptoms of cancer and its treatment.[76] The prevalence of cancer-related fatigue is not clear, but has been reported to be as high as 99%.[77] Fatigue leads to dramatic decrements in quality of life and overall performance status for many patients.[78] Studies of health-related quality of life identify pain, anxiety and fatigue as critically important symptoms.[84] The nearly universal nature of fatigue highlights the need for effective interventions, and to assess their potential impact on fatigue and quality of life. Most of the literature on asthenia is focused on the cancer patient, but many of the conclusions can be generalized to all patients with advanced chronic illness.

The pathophysiology of asthenia is not well understood. It has been postulated that asthenia has both neural and muscular origins. Further, there are two major neural types of fatigue: central and peripheral, with the peripheral type having two subtypes based upon proposed physiologic mechanisms–high-frequency (impaired action potential transmission/propagation) and low-frequency (impaired excitation-contraction coupling).[80]

The etiology of asthenia/fatigue is also not clearly understood, and is almost certainly multifactorial. In cancer, the tumor itself contributes to fatigue both from tumor burden[81] and from prolonged illness,[82] as well as other probable causes. Additionally, many of the anti-cancer therapies including chemotherapy, radiation therapy, and especially biologic response modifiers (Interferon-alpha) are known to cause fatigue. Anemia is a frequent occurrence in patients with advanced chronic diseases,[85] and has been shown to correlate with fatigue.[79] Additionally, malnutrition has been associated with fatigue.[78] Some claim that lactic acid accumulation and wasting of type II muscle fibers may be mechanisms for asthenic symptoms seen in advanced chronic illness.[74] Opioids have been questioned as to their potential role in fatigue, but Blesh et al. found that there was no significant correlation between fatigue and opioid dose. They did find, however, that increasing pain intensity was correlated with fatigue.[82] While steroids are often used beneficially to impact on many symptoms, they can also cause or exacerbate fatigue either from prolonged use causing myopathy or from their withdrawal. Infection, largely through release of cytokines, is also known to cause fatigue.

There are important psychological components to asthenia which are important to recognize. Piper et al. found a significant correlation between total fatigue and depression,[86] and Bruera et al. found a significant association between asthenia and psychological distress. This emphases the importance of the hospice interdisciplinary team in both the diagnosis and management of these complicated symptoms.

At present, there is no definitive therapy for fatigue. There is no evidence that aggressive nutritional correction in patients with advanced disease improves survival, improves quality of life[87] or impacts on fatigue.[88] Drugs that may cause or exacerbate asthenia should be discontinued. Steroids may be beneficial but the effect usually wanes in 4-8 weeks. Amphetamines such as methylphenidate have been shown to improve depressive symptoms fairly quickly,[89] increase energy levels[90] and may also directly or indirectly impact fatigue, though this has not been studied. Whether other impacts on psychological distress might impact fatigue (i.e., group therapy) is debated.[91]

Anemia is a frequent complication of cancer treatment and may result in a decrease in functional capacity and quality of life for patients. Erythropoetin alfa has been shown to increase hematocrit, decreases transfusion requirements, and produces significant improvements in energy, activity and overall quality of life. In fact, a direct correlation between improvement in quality of life and increased hemoglobin was observed in cancer patients treated with erythropoetin alfa.[79] Furthermore, recent data suggests that exercise positively impacts on fatigue.[78,83,92] Studies are currently underway to determine the benefits of a specific type of exercise–progressive resistance training (PRT)–with erythropoetin alfa in anemic cancer patients and PRT with megestrol. Other studies might consider the variable combinations of steroids/progestationals, PRT, methylphenidate and erythropoetin alfa. Clearly, this prevalent symptom complex is in need of further research to not only understand the pathophysiology, but to develop more effective means of treatment.

DELIRIUM AND TERMINAL AGITATION

One of the most widely feared consequences of terminal disease is loss of cognitive function and the subsequent loss of independence resulting from psychological as well as physical debility. Unfortunately, delirium, characterized by disturbances in arousal, awareness, perception, cognition and psychomotor behavior, is present in as many as 85% of terminally ill patients,[93,94] and results in increased distress for the patient, family and those who care for them. Delirium also complicates the evaluation and management of pain, dyspnea, nausea, anxiety and other problems common in terminally ill patients[95] and is probably a frequent contributing factor to terminal agitation and restlessness. To make matters worse, it is significantly underdiagnosed and undertreated.

There is, however, a growing consensus that early diagnosis and intervention can lead to significant patient improvement in this frequently reversible disorder.[96,97] As Wood and Ashby point out, the initial manifestations of delirium may be quite subtle, so clinical vigilance as well as sensitive and reliable screening tools are necessary.[98] While there are a number of tools available to screen for delirium and to assess cognitive function in general, the recently developed Memorial Delirium Assessment Scale is a concise and straightforward tool which specifically assesses symptom variability within a given day as well as to quantify its severity.[99] Further validation studies are needed, but it may prove to be very useful for patient care and research.

The etiology of delirium is usually complex in seriously ill patients, and includes such factors as infection, medications and their metabolites, dehydration, brain metastases, hypoxia, hypercalcemia and renal and hepatic dysfunction. Currently there is much interest in the potential contribution of opioids and their metabolites (specifically morphine, morphine-6-glucuronide and morphine-3-glucuronide) to neuropsychiatric dysfunction, especially in the context of renal insufficiency. While neither elevated plasma levels of M3G nor M6G (either in isolation or relative to total plasma morphine concentration) have been shown to definitively correlate with cognitive dysfunction,[98,100] ongoing inquiry in this area has led to the suggestion that opioids be rotated when cognitive dysfunction or overt delirium becomes manifest.[97,101,102]

Dehydration and the relative benefit of careful hydration (primarily to aid renal excretion of opioid and other metabolites) continues to be debated,[105-107] but a judicious trial of fluid resuscitation should be considered in the acutely delirious patient. Finally, after infectious and metabolic derangements have been addressed, opioid rotation has been initiated and hydration status has been assessed, the use of neuroleptic medications is a frequently overlooked and therefore underutilized intervention.[96] In a recent prospective, randomized, double-blind trial of hospitalized AIDS patients who developed delirium, Breitbart et al. found that both haloperidol and chlorpromazine helped to ameliorate the symptoms of delirium, and that chlorpromazine significantly improved cognitive functioning as measured by Folstein Mini-Mental State scores after 48 hours of treatment. Lorazepam alone was not effective and this part of the study was terminated early.[103]

It is clear that much remains to be clarified in the diagnosis and treatment of delirium. Consistent screening, early diagnosis and timely intervention can provide significant relief to seriously ill patients with delirium. For patients who are delirius and very close to death (terminal delirium), however, such interventions may be overly burdensome. For those who are severely agitated and who are unlikely to survive longer than 24 to 48 hours, those with irreversible major organ failure, and for whom the above-mentioned interventions are judged to be too burdensome, the use of benzodiazepines or sedating neuroleptics (such as chlorpromazine) to achieve "terminal sedation" remains the standard of care. This is an area ripe for further research.

DEPRESSION

Depression may occur in over half of terminally ill patients.[104] As with delirium, the diagnosis of major depression is problematic–not least because somatic manifestations of depression are central to the diagnosis. Furthermore, many of these symptoms can be attributed to their primary illness or its treatment and associated toxicities, rather than reflecting psychopathology. Yet accurate diagnosis and proper treatment remains important because depression, like delirium, profoundly impacts patients' quality of life, impairs their ability to significantly interact with family and caregivers, and complicates effective symptom control. It is also important to remember that depression is not an inevitable component of dying.

As Breitbart points out, it is important to distinguish between sadness and major depression, though this can prove challenging.[104] For patients without terminal disease, a personal or family history of depression is an important prognostic factor. In addition, increasing physical disability, advanced disease and pain have also been shown to be risk factors for depression.[108] Somatic manifestations of depression, such as fatigue, anorexia, sleep disturbances, can prove unreliable in the diagnosis of major depression in advanced disease. However, when symptoms seem to be out of proportion to a patient's stage of disease (and investigation has ruled out likely physical etiologies), or when a patient presents with a multitude of poorly defined and often intractable symptoms, the possibility of an underlying depression should be considered.[109] Hopelessness and anhedonia are key signs of depression, as most patients maintain the ability to experience pleasure in many aspects of daily life, even up to death.[108,110] This sense of hopefulness is maintained, even though its focus may change from hope for cure to hope for alleviation of discomfort, to hope for meaningful interactions with family and friends, to hope for a good dying. Persistent hopelessness is particularly ominous as it has been associated with an increased risk of suicide, particularly in those with advanced disease.[110] Yet despite all of this diagnostic complexity, Chochinov and colleagues remind us that a simple, single and often overlooked question may prove to be the most helpful: "Are you depressed?"[111]

With the exception of the advent of some new antidepressant medications, the treatment of depression has not evolved significantly over the past several years. Much depends on the patient's prognosis and their ability to participate in their care. For those who are likely to live for several weeks to months (or longer), brief psychotherapy, support groups, music and art therapy and relaxation techniques can often prove helpful. Pharmacologic therapy, however, remains fundamental, especially as an individual's physical condition deteriorates. The choice of medication is generally governed by the patient's prognosis (as the antidepressant action of some drugs may take several weeks to reach their full effect) and by the side effect profile. Tricyclic antidepressants, although effective, have the most bothersome side effects and are often not first line drugs, unless treating concomitant neuropathic pain. Newer agents such as selective serotonin reuptake inhibitors (paroxetine, fluoxetine, sertraline) and mixed neurotransmitter reuptake inhibitors (venlafaxine) have more favorable side effect profiles (but may still cause nausea, anorexia or a brief increase in anxiety) and have less potential for cardiac toxicity or other potentially life threatening complications of overdose. They may prove particularly helpful in depression associated with pancreatic cancer in which a serotonergic abnormality has been postulated, but this requires further study.[108] Other promising agents include mirtazepine and bupropion. For depressed patients who are unlikely to survive long enough to benefit from the above medications, or whose depression is serious enough to require immediate effects, psychostimulants such as methylphenidate, dextroamphetamine and pemoline can often prove helpful.[112-114] Improvement in mood and increased energy may occur within 24 hours. Prospective studies comparing the efficacy of these agents in depressed terminally ill patients would aid clinicians in choosing among the ever-increasing array of antidepressant medications.

In a recent study of patients with chronic pain, Sist and colleagues found that depressed patients reported not only an increased intensity of pain, but were significantly more likely to experience and to describe their pain using terms such as "fearful," "terrifying," "punishing," "cruel" and "killing."[115] Thus pain and depression seem to have a powerful and destructive synergy which profoundly increases the suffering of many patients. For this reason, developing and implementing more accurate diagnostic tools and therapeutic interventions in terminally ill patients is as essential as pain control and the management of nausea or dyspnea. Further investigation into that most elusive but vital phenomenon of hope is also essential, as it is an indispensable element of human well-being–not only for those suffering from terminal disease and depression, but for all of us.

REFERENCES

Neuropathic Pain

1. Martin L, Hagen N. (1997) Neuropathic pain in cancer patients: Mechanisms, Syndromes, and Clinical Controversies. *Journal of Pain and Symptom Management*; 14:99-117.

2. Portenoy R. (1998) Adjuvant analgesics in pain management. In: Doyle D, Hanks G, MacDonald N, eds. *The Oxford Textbook of Palliative Medicine.* Oxford: Oxford University Press, 361-390.

3. Portenoy R. (1998) Introduction: Neuropathic pain: From unresolved questions to clinical practice. In: Bruera E, Portenoy R, eds. *Topics in Palliative Care,* Volume 2, Oxford University Press, 3-5.

4. Max MB, Culnane M, Schafer SC et al. (1987) Amitriptyline relieves diabetic neuropathy pain in patients with normal or depressed mood. *Neurology,* 37:589-596.

5. Max MB, Kishore-Kumar R, Schafer SC et al. *(1991)* Efficacy of disipramine in painful diabetic neuropathy: a placebo controlled trial. *Pain*, 45:3-9.

6. Kishore-Kumar R, Max MB, Schafer SC et al. (1990) Desipramine relieves postherpetic neuralgia. *Journal of Clinical Pharmacology and Therapeutics*, 47:305-312.

7. Sindrup SH, Gram LF, Brosen K, Eshou O, Mogensen EF. (1990) The selective serotonin reuptake inhibitor paroxetine is effective in the treatment of diabetic neuropathy symptoms. *Pain* 42:135-144.

8. Rull JA, Quibrera R, Gonzalez-Millan H, te al. (1969) Symptomatic treatment of peripheral diabetic neuropathy with carbamazepine: double blind crossover trial. *Diabetologia*, 5:215-220.

9. Swerdlow M, Cundill JG. (1981) Anticonvulsant drugs used in the treatment of lancinating pains. A comparison. *Anesthesia*, 36:1129-1132.

10. Mellick GA, Mellick LB. (1995) Gabapentin in the management of reflex sympathetic dystrophy (letter). *Journal of Pain and Symptom Management*, 10:265-266.

11. Wetzel CH, Connelly JF. (1997) Use of gabapentin in pain management. *The Annals of Pharmacotherapy*; 31:1082-1083.

12. Rosner H, Rubin L, Kestenbaum A. (1996) Gabapentin adjuctive therapy in neuropathic pain states. *Clinical Journal of Pain*, 12:56-58.

13. Fromm GH, Terence CF, Chattha AS. (1984) Baclofen in the treatment of trigeminal neuralgia: double-blind study and long-term follow-up. *Annals of Neurology*, 15:240-244.

14. Fromm GH. (1994) Baclofen as an adjuvant analgesic. *Journal of Pain and Symptom Management*, 9:500-509.

15. Gobelet C, Waldburger M, Meier JL. (1992) The effect of adding calcitonin to physical treatment on reflex sympathetic dystrophy. *Pain* 48:171-175.

16. Bruera E, Ripamonti C, Brenneis C, Macmillan K, Hanson J. (1992) A randomized double-blind crossover trial of intravenous lidocaine in the treatment of neuropathic cancer pain. *Journal of Pain and Symptom Management* 7:138-140.

17. Kastrup J, Petersen P, Dejgard A, Angelo HR, Hilsted J. (1987) Intravenous lidocaine infusion-a new treatment of chronic painful neuropathy? *Pain* 28:69-75.

18. Brose WG, Cousins MJ. (1991) Subcutaneous lidocaine for treatment of neuropathic cancer pain. *Pain* 45:145-148.

19. Dejgard A, Petersen P, Kastrup J. (1988) Mexiletine for treatment of chronic painful diabetic neuropathy. *Lancet* I:9-11.

20. Curatolo M, Petersen-Felix S, Arendt-Nielsen L, Zbinden A. (1997) Epidural epinephrine and clonidine. *Anesthesiology* 87:785-794.

21. Eisenach J, DuPen S, Dubois M, Miguel R, Allin D. (1995) Epidural clonidine analgesia for intractable cancer pain. *Pain* 61:391-399.

22. Yang C, Wong C, Chang J, Ho S. (1996) Intrathecal ketamine reduces morphine requirements in patients with terminal cancer pain. *Canadian Journal of Anaesthesia* 43:379-383.

23. Mercadante S, Lodi F, Sapio M, Calligara M, Serretta R. (1995) Long-term ketamine subcutaneous continuous infusion in neuropathic cancer pain. *Journal of Pain and Symptom Management* 10:564-568.

24. Clark J, Kalan G. (1995) Effective treatment of severe cancer pain of the head using low-dose ketamine in an opioid-tolerant patient. *Journal of Pain and Symptom Management* 10:310-314.

25. Kinnman E, Nygards E, Hansson P. (1997) Effects of dextromethorphan in clinical doses on capsaicin-induced ongoing pain and mechanical hypersensitivity. *Journal of Pain and Symptom Management* 14:195-201.

26. Ebert B, Andersen S, Hjeds H, Dickenson A. (1998) Dextropropoxyphene acts as a noncomptetitive N-methyl-D-aspartate antagonist. *Journal of Pain and Symptom Management* 15:269-274.

27. Pud D, Eisenberg E, Spitzer A et al. (1998) The NMDA receptor antagonist amantadine reduces surgical neuropathic pain in cancer patients: a double-blind, randomized, placebo-controlled trial. *Pain* 75:349-354.

Dyspnea

28. Ahmedzai S. (1998) Palliation of respiratory symptoms. In: D Doyle, GWC Hanks, & N MacDonald, eds. *Oxford Textbook of Palliative Medicine.* Oxford: Oxford University Press 9.5, pp 583-616.

29. Bruera E, Neumann CM. (1998) Management of specific symptom complexes. *Canadian Medical Association Journal* 158 (13): 1717-1726.

30. Bruera E, Ripamonti C. (1998) Dyspnea in patients with advanced cancer. In: AM Berger, RK Portenoy, & DE Weissman, eds. *Principles and Practice of Supportive Oncology.* Philadelphia: Lippincott-Raven Publishers, 295-308

31. Bruera E, Ripamonti C. (1997) Dyspnea: Pathophysiology and Assessment. *Journal of Pain and Symptom Management* (13)4: 220-232.

32. Neely K, Krammer L. (1998) End of life care: Palliative strategies for vomiting and dyspnea. *Family Practice Recertification* (20) 6: 13-40.

33. Hay L, Farncombe M, McKee P. (1996) Patient, nurse and physician views of dyspnea. *Cancer Nurse* 92:26-29.

34. Bruera E, Kuehn N, Miller MJ et al. (1991) The Edmonton symptom assessment system (ESAS): a simple method for the assessment of palliative care patients. *Journal of Palliative Care* 7:6-9.

35. Farcombe M, Chater S, Gillis A. (1994) The use of nebulised opioids for breathlessness: a chart review. *Palliative Medicine* 8:306-312.

36. Davis C. (1995) The role of nebulised drugs in palliating respiratory symptoms of malignant disease. *European Journal of Palliative Care* 2: 9-15.

37. Bruera E, MacEachern T, Ripamonti C et al. (1993) Subcutaneous morphine for dyspnea in cancer patients. *Annals of Int Med* 119:906-907.

38. Tobin MJ. (1990) Dyspnea: Pathopysiologic basis, clinical presentation, and management. *Archives of Internal Medicine* 150: 1604-1612.

Constipation/Diarrhea

39. Sykes, NP. (1993) Constipation and diarrhea. In: D. Doyle, GWC Hanks, & N. MacDonald, eds. *Oxford Textbook of Palliative Medicine.* Oxford: Oxford University Press 4.4:513-526.

40. Fallon M, O'Neill B. (1997) Constipation and diarrhea. *British Medical Journal* 315: 1293-1296.

41. Mercande S. (1998) Diarrhea, malabsorption and constipation. In: A. Berger, R.K. Portenoy, & D.E. Weismann, eds. *Principles and Practice of Supportive Oncology*. Philadelphia: Lippincott-Raven Publishers 191-206.

42. Burke A. (1994) The management of constipation in end-stage disease. *Australian Family Physician* 23: 1248-1253.

43. Sykes NP. (1994) Current approaches to the management of constipation. *Cancer Surveys* 21: 137-145.

Nausea/Vomiting

44. Fainsinger R, Miller M, Bruera E, Hanson J, Maceachern T. (1991) Symptom control during the last week of life on a palliative care unit. *Journal of Palliative Care*, 7:5-11.

45. Kinghorn S. (1997) Palliative Care: Nausea and vomiting. *Nursing Times* 93;57-60.

46. Vaino A, Auvinen A. (1996) Prevalence of symptoms among patients with advanced cancer: An international collaborative study. *Journal of Pain and Symptom Management* 12:3-10.

47. Mannix KA. (1993) Palliation of nausea and vomiting. In: D Doyle, GWC Hanks, & N MacDonald, eds. *Oxford Textbook of Palliative Medicine*. Oxford: Oxford University Press 9.3, 489-499.

48. Fallon BG. (1998) Nausea and vomiting unrelated to cancer treatment. In: AM Berger, RK Portenoy, & DE Weissman, eds. *Principles and Practice of Supportive Oncology*. Philadelphia: Lippincott-Raven Publishers 179-189.

49. Pisters KMW, Kris M. (1998) Treatment related nausea and vomiting. In: AM Berger, RK Portenoy, & DE Weissman, eds. *Principles and Practice of Supportive Oncology*. Philadelphia: Lippincott-Raven Publishers, 165-177.

50. Baines, MJ. (1997) Nausea, vomiting and intestinal obstruction. *British Medical Journal* 315: 1148-1150.

51. Lichter I. (1993) Results of antiemetic management in terminal illness. *Journal of Palliative Care* 9:19-21.

Intestinal Obstruction

52. Baines, MJ. (1998) Malignant Intestinal Obstruction. In: D. Doyle, GWC Hanks, & N. MacDonald, eds. Oxford Textbook of Palliative Medicine. Oxford: *Oxford University Press* 9.3.4, pp 531.

53. Storey, PS. (1991) Obstruction of the GI tract. *Am. J. Hospice and PC*, May/June pg.5.

54. Aranha, GV et al. (1981) Surgical palliation of small bowel obstruction due to metastatic carcinoma. *Am Surgeon*, 47:99-102.

55. DeConno, F et al. (1991) The continuous subcutaneous infusion of hyoscine butylbromide reduces secretions in patients with gastrointestinal obstruction. *J Pain and Symptom Management*, 6:484-6.

56. Hutchison, SMW et al. (1995) Increased serotonin excretion in patients with ovarian carcinoma and intestinal obstruction. *Palliative Medicine*, 9:67-8.

57. Fallon, MT, (1996) The physiology of somatostatin and its synthetic analog, octreotide. *Eu. J. Pall Care*, 1(1): 20-22.

58. Lamberts SWJ et al. *(1995) Drug therapy: Octreotide. New Eng J Med* 334:4 246-254.

Anorexia-Cachexia

59. Puccio M, Nathanson L. (1997) The cancer cachexia syndrome. *Sem in Oncol* 24(3):277-278.

60. Dewys WD et al. (1980) Prognostic effect of weight loss prior to chemotherapy in cancer patients. Eastern Cooperative Oncology Group. *Am J of Med* 69(4):491-7.

61. Bruera E. (1997) ABC of palliative care. Anorexia, cachexia and nutrition. *BMJ* 315(7117):1219-1222.

62. Techekmedyian NS, Heber D. (1993) Cancer and AIDS cachexia: mechanisms and approach to therapy. *Oncology* 7:55-59.

63. Beal JE. (1995) Dronabinol as treatment for anorexia associated weight loss in patients with fatigue. *J Pain and Symptom Management* 10:89-97.

64. Wadleigh R et al. (1990) Dronabinol enhancement of appetite in 5 cancer patients. *Proc Am Clin Oncol* 9:1280.

65. Nelson KA et al. (1994) A phase II study of delta-9-tetrahydrcannabinol for appetite stimulation in cancer associated anorexia. *J Pall Care* 10:14-19.

66. Kardinal CG, Loprinzi CL, Schaid DJ et al. (1990) A controlled trial of cyproheptadine cancer patients with anorexia and/or cachexia. *Cancer* 65: 2657-2662.

67. Loprinzi CL, Kuross SA, O'Fallon JR et al. (1994) Randomized placebo controlled evaluation of hydrazine sulfate in patients with advanced colorectal cancer. *J Clin Oncol* 12: 1126-1129.

68. Goldberg RM, Loprinzi Cl, Maillard JA et al. (1995) Pentoxifylline for treatment of cancer anorexia and cachexia? A randomized, double blind, placebo controlled trial. *J Clin Oncol* 13: 2856-2859.

69. Tchekmedyian NS, Tait N, Moody M et al. (1987) High dose megestrol acetate: A possible treatment for cachexia. *JAMA* 9: 1195-1198.

70. Loprinzi CL, Ellison NM, Schaid DJ et al. (1990) Controlled trial of megestrol acetate for the treatment of cancer anorexia and cachexia. *J Natl Cancer Inst* 82: 1127-1132.

71. Loprinzi CL, Michalak JC, Schaid DJ et al. (1993) Phase III evaluation of four doses of megestrol acetate as therapy for patients with cancer anorexia and/or cachexia. *J of Clin Oncol* 11: 762-767.

72. Loprinzi CL, Schaid DJ, Dose AM et al. (1993) Body composition changes in patients who gain weight while receiving megestrol acetate. *J Clin Oncol* 11: 152-154.

Asthenia/Fatigue

73. Rowland LP, Schotland DL. (1965) Neoplasms and Muscle Disease. In: Brain WR, Norris FH, eds. *The remote effects of cancer on the nervous system.* New York: Grune and Stratton, 83-97.

74. Theologides A. (1982) Asthenia in cancer. *Am J Med* 73:1-3.

75. Bruera E, MacDonald RN. (1988) Asthenia in patients with advanced cancer. Issues in symptom control. Part I, *J Pain and Symptom Managment* 3(4):211.

76. Ferrell BR et al. (1996) Bone Tired: The experience of fatigue and its impact on quality of life. *Onc Nurs For* 23(10):1539-1547.

77. Messias DK et al. (1997) Patients' perspectives of fatigue while undergoing chemotherapy. *Onc Nurs For 24*(1):43-48.

78. Winningham ML et al. (1994) Fatigue and the cancer experience: The state of the knowledge. *Onc Nurs For* 21(1):23-36.

79. Glaspy J et al. (1998) Impact of therapy with epoetin alfa on clinical outcomes in patients with nonmyeloid malignancies during cancer chemotherapy in community oncology practice. *J Clin Oncol* 15(3):1218-1234.

80. Sahlin K (1994) Acid-base balance during high intensity exercise. In: Harries, Williams, Stanish, Micheli, eds. *Oxford Textbook of Sports Medicine.* New York: Oxford University Press; 45-52.

81. Pickard-Holley S. (1991) Fatigue in cancer patients. A descriptive study. *Cancer Nursing* 14:13-19.

82. Blesch KS, Paice JA, Wickham R et al. (1991) Correlates of fatigue in people with breast or lung cancer. *Oncology Nurs Forum* 18:81-87.

83. Freindenreich CM, Courneya KS. (1996) Exercise as rehabilitation for cancer patients. *Clin J Sport Med* 6(4):237-44.

84. Neuenschwander H, Bruera E. (1998) Asthenia. In: Doyle D, Hanks G, MacDonald N, eds. *Oxford Textbook of Palliative Medicine.* New York: Oxford University Press; 573.

85. Skillings JR, Shridar FG, Wong C (1993) The frequency of red cell transfusion for anemia in patients receiving chemotherapy: a retrospective cohort study. *Am J Clin Oncol* 16:22-25.

86. Piper BF et al. (1989) The development of an instrument to measure the subjective dimension of fatigue. In: Funk, SG et al. eds. *Key aspects of comfort: management of pain, fatigue and nausea.* New York: Springer-Verlag; 199-208.

87. Bruera E, Fainsinger RL. (1993) Clinical management of cachexia and anorexia. In: Doyle, D, Hanks, G, MacDonald, N, eds. *Oxford Textbook of Palliative Medicine.* New York: Oxford University Press; 330-337.

88. Nelson KA, Walsh D, Sheehan FA. (1993) The cancer anorexia-cachexia syndrome. *J Clin Oncol* 16:22-25.

89. Gurian B, Rosowsky E. (1990) Lowdose methylphenidate in the very old. *J of Ger Psychiatry & Neurology,* 3(3):152-4.

90. Bruera E, Chadwick S, Brenneis C. (1985) Methylphenidate associated with narcotics for the treatment of cancer pain. *Cancer Treat Rep* 70:295-297.

91. Bruera E, Portenoy R eds. (1998) *Topics in Palliative Care.* Volume 2. New York: Oxford University Press; 195-202.

92. Singh NA, Clements KM, Fiatarone MA, (1997) A randomized controlled trial of progressive resistance training in depressed elders. *J Gerontol* 52A(1); M27-35.

Delirium

93. Breitbart W, Bruera E, Harvey C, Lynch (1995) M. Neuropsychiatric syndromes and psychological symptoms in patients with advanced cancer. *Journal of Pain and Symptom Management* 10:131-141.
94. Massie MJ, Holland J, Glass E. (1983) Delirium in terminally ill cancer patients. *Am J of Psychiatry* 140:1048-1050.
95. Coyle N, Breitbart W, Weaver S, Portenoy R. (1994) Delirium as a contributing factor to "crescendo" pain: three case reports. *Journal of Pain and Symptom Management* 9:44-47.
96. MacDonald N. (1995) Suffering and dying in cancer patients–Research frontiers in controlling confusin, cachexia, and dyspnea. In: Caring for Patients at the End of Life (special issue). *Western Journal of Medicine* 163:278-286.
97. Pereira J, Hanson J, Bruera E. (1997) The frequency and clinical course of cognitive impairment in patients with terminal cancer. *Cancer* 79:835-842.
98. Wood M, Ashby M, Somogyi A, Fleming B. (1998) Neuropsychological and pharmacokinetic assessment of hospice inpatients receiving morphine. *Journal of Pain and Symptom Management* 16:112-120.
99. Breitbart W, Rosenfeld B, Roth A, Smith M, Cohen K, Passik S. (1997) The Memorial Delirium Assessment Scale. *Journal of Pain and Symptom Management* 13:128-137.
100. Tiseo P, Thaler H, Lapin J, Inturrisi C, Portenoy R, Foley K. (1995) Morphine-6-glucuronide concentrations and opioid-related side effects: a survey in cancer patients. *Pain* 61:47-54.
101. Bruera E, Franco J, Maltoni M, Watanabe S, Suarez-Almazor M. (1995) Changing pattern of agitated impairental status in patients with advanced cancer: association with cognitive monitoring, hydration, and opioid rotation. *Journal of Pain and Symptom Management* 10:287-291.
102. DeStoutz N, Bruera E, Suarez-Almazor M. (1995) Opioid rotation for toxicity reduction in terminal cancer patients. *Journal of Pain and Symptom Management* 10:378-384.
103. Breitbart W, Marotta R, Platt M, Weisman H et al. (1996) A double-blind trial of haloperidol, chlorpromazine, and lorazepam in the treatment of delirium in hospitalized AIDS patients. *American Journal of Psychiatry* 153:231-237.

Depression

104. Breitbart W, Bruera E, Chochinov H, Lynch M. (1995) Neuropsychiatric syndromes and psychological symptoms in patinets with advanced cancer. *Journal of Pain and Symptom Management* 10:131-141.
105. Fainsinger RL, Bruera E. (1997) When to treat dehydration in the terminally ill? *Supportive Care in Cancer* 5(3):205-11.

106. Fainsinger RL, MacEachern T, Miller MJ, Bruera E et al. (1994) The use of hypodermoclysis for rehydration in terminally ill cancer patients. *J Pain and Symptom Management*, 9:298-302.

107. Dunphy K, Finlay N, Rathbone G et al. (1995) Rehydration in palliative medicine and terminal care: if not-why not? *Palliative Medicine* 9:221-8.

108. Passik S, Breitbart W. (1996) Depression in patients with pancreatic carcinoma. Cancer 78:615-626.

109. Barraclough J. (1997) Depression, anxiety, and confusion. *British Medical Journal* 315:1365-1368.

110. Chochinov H, Wilson K, Enns M, Lander S. (1998) Depression, hopelessness, and suicidal ideation in the terminally ill. *Psychosomatics* 39:366-370.

111. Chochinov H, Wilson K, Enns M, Lander S. (1997) "Are you depressed?" Screening for depression in the terminally ill. *American Journal of Psychiatry* 154:674-676.

112. Breitbart W, Chochinov M, Passik S. (1998) Psychiatric aspects of palliative care. In: Doyle D, Hanks G, MacDonald N, eds. *Oxford Textbook of Palliative Medicine*. Oxford: Oxford University Press.

113. Fernandez F, Adams F, Holmes V et al. (1987) Methylphenidate for depressive disorders in cancer patients. *Psychosomatics* 28:455-461.

114. Burns M, Eisendrath S. (1994) Dextroamphetamine treatment for depression in terminally ill patients. *Psychosomatics* 35:80-82.

115. Sist T, Florio G, Miner M, Lema M, Zevon M. (1998) The relationship between depression and pain language in cancer and chronic non-cancer pain patients. *Journal of Pain and Symptom Management* 15:350-358.

Spirituality

Emily Chandler

SUMMARY. At the present time, there is a widening search for spirituality as distinct from organized religion, particularly as it relates to well-being, wholeness, and healing. In both professional and lay contexts, spirituality has come to the forefront of public consciousness. The place of spirituality within the hospice movement is not unaffected by this shift in popular priorities. Once the prerogative of chaplains and clergy, the nurturing of spiritual journeys is now becoming a common concern. Experiencing *sensory spirituality* can provide both caregivers and those for whom they care a blessed respite for bodies, minds, and spirits. *[Article copies available for a fee from The Haworth Document Delivery Service: 1-800-342-9678. E-mail address: getinfo@haworthpressinc.com <Website: http://www.haworthpressinc.com>]*

INTRODUCTION

No other human experience encompasses such a range of emotions for the patient and his or her world than that of dying. Witnessing and contemplating the unknown, we are all confronted with feelings of hopelessness as well as hope, sadness as well as peace, and fear as well as trust. All of us wonder about the mystery that extends our reach. Perhaps more than any other human experience, the hope of life after life, or even the fear of its absence, launches a spiritual journey.

Often that journey is hampered by old experiences; memories from childhood that confuse rather than enlighten, that hurt instead of heal. Spiritual journeys are distinct from religious belief in that they involve

[Haworth co-indexing entry note]: "Spirituality." Chandler, Emily. Co-published simultaneously in *The Hospice Journal* (The Haworth Press, Inc.) Vol. 14, No. 3/4, 1999, pp. 63-74; and: *The Hospice Heritage: Celebrating Our Future* (ed: Inge B. Corless and Zelda Foster) The Haworth Press, Inc., 1999, pp. 63-74. Single or multiple copies of this article are available for a fee from The Haworth Document Delivery Service [1-800-342-9678, 9:00 a.m. - 5:00 p.m. (EST). E-mail address: getinfo@haworthpressinc.com].

us in the mystery of *experiencing* the holy, the mysterious. Nourishing the inward journey with available and accessible *sensory* spirituality, opens up new possibilities of awareness as we explore expressions of the sacred. At the present time, there is a widening search for spirituality as distinct from organized religion, particularly in regard to healing (Colt, 1996; Cousineau, 1995; Samuels, 1995; Wallis, 1996). There is ample evidence that spirituality enhances well-being in a variety of contexts, regardless of the definition of the term (Burton, 1998; Fehring, Miller, & Shaw, 1997; Koenig, 1995; Koenig et al., 1992; Matthews et al., 1998; Mickley, Soeken, & Belcher, 1992).

Spirituality in its many forms and varieties of experience has had a central place in the hospice movement since its inception, although in the American tradition we have been less self-consciously involved than our British counterparts (Millison, 1995). The mandate to include spiritual care as a benefit of hospice has preceded our cultural inclinations; in many instances we were providing spiritual care as a pragmatic necessity rather than as a perceived need. While there has been pressure to bring the rigors of research to the issue of spirituality (McGrath, 1997), the area is cluttered with philosophical issues, political concerns, and pragmatic realities. And we can't seem to come to consensus on a definition of either terms, or usage. Confusion exists within, never-mind between, professions as well as cultures (Babler, 1997; Dyson, Cobb, & Forman, 1997; Emblen, 1992; Halstead & Mickley, 1997; Martsolf, 1997; Macrae, 1995).

It is not the purpose here to resolve those dilemmas; that effort requires a tour de force beyond the scope of this essay. Rather, the course that spiritual journeys themselves seem to take will be the focus–with a closer look at the affective concomitants of the process, as opposed to the impact of cognitive belief.

SPIRITUAL JOURNEYS

Revisiting the course journeys take can be helpful in guiding our thinking about spiritual journeys. What has been classically known as the hero/heroine's journey, refers to stories of transformation that are usually divided into three distinct stages or sections, much like a three act play; there is a beginning, a middle, and an end. Joseph Campbell delineates the process as the mythic adventure of the hero: departure, initiation, and return (Campbell, (1968). In Biblical images, this marginalized time of wandering recalls images of the desert, the wilderness, images of lostness and not knowing. It also holds out the promise of new life.

The phases of the journey that lead from old ways of being to the new, can be described as incorporating the attendant elements of grief; denial, anger, bargaining, chaos, depression, resignation, openness, readiness, and re-emergence (Perlman & Takacs, 1990). Those phenomena reflect the three-fold process to which Campbell (1968) refers:

1. loss of structure   (denial, anger, bargaining)
2. chaos: into the woods   (chaos, depression, resignation)
3. re-structuring   (openness, readiness, re-emergence)

The beginning of the journey always consists of some kind of leave-taking; leaving home, or some *loss of structure* that previously provided the order of life, the boundary lines of one's universe. The impact of loss is generally felt as one moves out of the familiar into the next phase of the journey. The transition within the transition, the movement away from one phase to another, becomes a microcosm of the way grief is encountered. Avoiding the pain of transition at this first juncture sets the stage for a trajectory of avoidance as a method of coping that can begin to take on a life of its own. It is critically important to be able to sit with the emptiness, the pain of loneliness, separation anxiety, confusion, and bewilderment. Loss of structure with attendant feelings of denial, anger, and bargaining can truncate the spiritual journey from the beginning. It's much easier to tolerate the aching absence of feeling if there is a viable alternative offering hope. Hope in this context implies promise of redemption, renewal, and resurrection; the hope that some phoenix will indeed rise up from these ashes of sadness, frustration, and disappointment.

This is the place where it is essential to nurture, to nourish the hungry soul with real spiritual food, not toxic faith or empty religiosity that is nothing more than an imitation of spirituality, and poisonous to the life of the spirit. Here we need vibrant images of faith as we search for the face of God, sounds of comfort and joy as we strain to hear if there does exist a still, small voice. Here we need hope of the promised land, as we wander in the wilderness of the desert. There's always a tendency to bypass the work of the desert–and go racing toward Canaan. There's always the possibility of mistaking sensation for feeling, efficiency for order, law for ethics, legalism for morality, or illusion for apprehension.

Sitting with the pain implies waiting in the desert, wandering in the wilderness, getting lost in the woods. Discovering what to do while one's waiting becomes the stuff of which real art is fashioned; the senses, perhaps for want of anything else, become engaged in the in-between time. When all we are is all we have–we create. We paint, we sing, we pray, we sculpt, we dance, we write poetry, we tell stories. Uncovering ways to mobilize creativity and passion out of a spiritual center is at the heart of this healing time.

This is the time for a holding community that can provide "good enough" support, good enough counseling, good enough re-membering, good enough spiritual care. At this juncture we need images, metaphors, symbols, rituals, and stories that that can point beyond themselves, that are capable of carrying the weight of unseen hope. Patients and families suffering from dis-ease that is related to their spirits as well as their bodies may have no language with which to ask their questions. They need spirituality presented in a manner their hearts can understand; experiential as well as cognitive, relational as well as rational. Activating hope is central to the task.

The movement toward holistic care is pushing healers from multiple disciplines to examine their own presuppositions regarding healing and wholeness and to examine their own wholeness as well. It is only when one has undertaken one's own spiritual journey that the paths of others' journeys become discernible. What has been understood to be "burnout" characterized by withdrawal, depression, anger, and stress may really be post-traumatic stress disorder, or spiritual distress in the caregiver. Given the pressure and pace of the current situation in hospice care, this need for centeredness in one's own spiritual life is even more critical.

It has long been demonstrated that so-called "secondary victimization" occurs in professionals and people who witness trauma on a regular basis: clergy, therapists, police, emergency medical technicians, emergency room personnel, firefighters and, of course, hospice staff. Hearing the stories, witnessing the grief, may result in a mirror image of those symptoms in care-givers over time. Psychic numbing, that hallmark of PTSD, can be masked as depression, burnout, disinterest, ineffectiveness, hostility, or even sexual misconduct (Chandler, 1993). But those whom we call burned out or depressed may, in fact, be disspirited. The holding of painful stories, of grief, sadness and despair, puts the caregiver at risk for development of physical disease as well; there is considerable evidence to suggest that many physical problems, from allergies to the development of cancer occur when people are susceptible, or more specifically, immunosuppresed. For victims to become survivors, and healers to themselves become healed, an accessible and fitting spiritual life than can support wholeness and renewal is essential. We who profess to be the healers of the spirit may first need to be healed ourselves.

It is not hard to imagine the stress that resides in the hearers of the stories of trauma, pain, and distress. Symptoms are intensified when the individual is exposed to situations, activities that resemble or symbolize the original trauma. Uncovering a repertoire of healing triggers that are more powerful than the painful triggers that precipitate a traumatic response is essential. Otherwise, we are all in danger of becoming so numb that we ourselves become victimizers of those whose pain we would alleviate, simply because the tears are too hard to watch, the story too difficult to hear. Yet it is precisely in hearing the stories of spiritual journeys, which are often filled with suffering and chaos, that both the teller and the hearer are transformed (Simpkinson & Simpkinson, 1993; Taylor, 1997). Storytelling and storyholding are themselves the activity that harbors the promise of hope: in the telling of the story, we begin to uncover the possibility of reframing what we see.

Protecting one's self against unbearable feelings of pain and loss can lead to a preference for cognitive ways of being as well as doing, especially for those who are exposed to extraordinary levels of stress, suffering, and grief. When one cannot tolerate the pain, reverting to intellectualization provides a way of "keeping an even keel." That then becomes the very antithesis of what is required for a spiritual connection or even an empathic human connection. The only way to break through the numbing that prevents feeling is to recognize the images, symbols, metaphors, rituals that are capable of creative, healing expression.

It is here that a repertoire of strategies to counteract the triggers of incapacitating feelings of grief and pain play an essential role in our ability to be helpful. Moving out of the lostness of the dark night of the soul, the wandering in the woods of chaos, requires the development of a spiritual life that is full and richly experiential. Sensory spirituality is accessed through what we see, hear, taste, touch and smell. The current resurgence of interest in alternative medicine and complementary modalities may reflect a growing poverty of nurturing sensory experience as well as a trend toward less invasive forms of medical treatment (Astin, 1998). In 1993, Eisenberg et al. reported a study of the use of "unconventional medical practices" in the United States. The results showed that fully one third of the population of the United States was using alternative therapies, or complementary modalities, and they were paying out of pocket: 10 billion dollars a year. Those who were using the modalities–from therapeutic touch and biofeedback to herbal medicine and aromatherapy–were clearly taking their well-being into their own hands. A recent follow-up study has shown a significant increase in the use of complementary modalities. In both studies, use of "self-prayer" was included as a question, although the results were excluded in the analysis. In fact there was a marked increase in the use of prayer from 25% in 1990, to 35% in 1997 (Eisenberg et al., 1998).

INTEGRATING SPIRITUALITY, THE ARTS, AND COMPLEMENTARY MODALITIES

"The soul," Thomas Moore tells us, "is always searching for itself and it takes great pleasure when it finds itself mirrored in the material world" (1996, p. 198). Sensory changes accompanying illness rob patients of positive experiences in their bodies, where the body is often their enemy. Employing the sensory experience the arts provide could make some part of the body their ally once again. And, given the diminishing sensory capacity of the dying, the synesthetic effect of using more than one form of expression is critical. Music, or sculpture, or art, or dance, or poetry can give expression to the urge toward spiritual yearning that may not even be sensed–let alone articulated. Using music and art with patients about to undergo surgery, for example, or with patients who are confused or in pain, particularly those who are dying, promotes a peaceful environment, and lessens feeling of anxiety and fear (Bailey, 1994; Beck, 1991; Hanser & Thompson, 1994; Whitcomb, 1993).

Chronic illness, pain, and increased attention to the process of dying has brought into focus the role of the arts for wholeness and healing. The arts can play a central, even critical role in expressing feeling and instilling hope. Engaging the arts in the service of relieving pain, enhancing wellness, and communicating feelings of well-being and peace has become increasingly important as people face questions of life and death (Bertman, 1994). A return to shamanistic respect for other, for the environment, and for the embodiment of soul is providing a significant countervalent force against cold, mechanistic technology. Our very ability to advance has precipitated an equal and opposite reaction; to engage the arts in the pursuit of spiritual wholeness and healing.

Sallie Bailey is a UCC clergywoman who uses music with hospice patients who are nearing the end of life. She is convinced that when people can access their creativity as a means of expression, they are best able to express feeling, pain, rage, fear–and then move on in the journey. Accessing feeling is best accomplished by the creative Spirit; people are enlivened through engagement with their art form.

> We receive images and sounds from the environment through the senses of our bodies. The images are processed through our emotions, spirit and mind and become inspirations/ideas that move through the body and are given form in other images and sounds. Thus, through the creative process, connections to each dimension of one's self are made. (Bailey, p. 329)

In Missola, Montana, *The Chalice of Repose* trains musicians to play the Celtic harp and sing in the presence of patients and families when death is imminent (Schroeder-Sheker, 1994). It is perhaps the happy congruence of comprehension and sensory or sensual feeling that constitutes an experience we refer to as soulful, or soul-making. We *know*, more than we can express, and we know in the inner recesses of our beings.

The dying, in particular, have changing sensory function that may constrict their devotional life, spiritual experience, or experience of the holy. In identifying the symbolic forms and archetypes that are apt to reinforce one position or feeling over and against another, we can be selective and intentional about forms that facilitate expression of feeling. Just as older adults, who know loss of friends and family, work and relevance, also know loss of hearing, sight, taste, and touch and smell, patients who are dying know how the loss of bodily, sensory function diminishes their lives. Nourishing the inward journey, with available and accessible sensory spirituality, opens up new possibilities of awareness and appreciation of life.

PSYCHOSOCIOSPIRITUAL CARE

A growing number of people are advocating the use of alternative modalities in bringing people to a more holistic way of being (Acterberg, Dossey, & Kolkmeier, 1994; Brown-Saltzman, 1997; Dossey, 1993). The complementary modalities which have been grouped under "alternative medicine" include acupuncture, therapeutic touch, biofeedback, relaxation, guided imagery, aromatherapy, chiropractic, herbal medicine, massage, and prayer. Dossey specifically elaborated his views with examples of what he calls non-local prayer, citing as his research base a number of studies using scientific protocols. Other researchers continue that effort (Levin, 1996; Levin, Lyons & Larson, 1994). Kathleen Fischer (1995), writing out of a more self-conscious spiritual perspective, is drinking from the same well. Her notions of healing interventions with women in the second half of life are borne out of her conviction that women's experience, imagination, embeddedness, connectedness, stories and images are their most viable source of spiritual sustenance. She offers rituals, insights, and observations about actualizing the redemptive power of spirituality for women who are undergoing change and transition, including loss.

Bereavement itself may initiate a search for the spirit. Family members who are taking care of parents, taking care of children, saying good-bye to both, and often finding themselves facing dreams deferred, may be more ready for the spiritual journey in to the depths of the self. They are often tired, depleted, wounded, empty, dry–and yearning for refreshment and renewal. The situation may lead both men and women to the same crossroads, although for different reasons. Men may not have had the inclination to make the spiritual journey; women have not had the time. Families facing transitional periods fraught with bereavement and grief need more than cognitive assurance, and even something more than a relational approach, although a relational context is critical. The only way to break through numbing to access the healing power of feeling, is to utilize the images, rituals, stories, music, and arts that can break through the wall of silence that weariness and grief erects–and touch the center of the soul.

Patients and families respond to the resources of the arts in different ways; identifying an individual's proclivity for taking in the holy is essential to this task. Attention to the particular senses that are especially operative for a given individual helps to make use of creative expression intentional, and therefore more efficacious. Using the senses as a starting point, the arts are easily employed in rituals, or exercises that give people an opportunity to express themselves and discover-or uncover their deepest spiritual yearnings. We can create opportunities to concretize symbols and rituals that are imbued with spiritual healing. Candles, incense, music, art, prayer, and guided imagery are all ways that the implicit can be made explicit, so that feelings are brought to life (Fischer, 1995; Thompson, 1995).

An act as simple as lighting a candle can be powerful. So can a container for tissues filled with tears-a small ritual that holds the hurt-and makes the tears in some small way, sacred. Intentional use of synesthesia, utilizing more than one sense at a time, enhances spiritual experience. Combining sights and sounds, for example, or sounds and aromas, powerfully reinforces healing memories.

As people committed to spiritual care, we need to create sacred space for patients, invite them to share their story, and provide a way for them to put down the burden of pain. It is in the creating, in sending the pain out into the universe, that both ourselves and our burdens are changed. When the stories are told, heard, honored, and grieved, something redemptive happens. What had been a source of pain and death becomes the genesis of new life in music, art, writing, dance, sculpting, film, poetry, sewing, woodwork, gardening. The old is finished and gone. Everything becomes fresh and new, as we fine tune the instrument of grace.

Hospice programs have provided what most people wish: managed pain, comfort, quality of life and a peaceful death. Experience with hospice has taught us that rather than being a fearful, dreadful experience, dying can be healing, peaceful, even spiritually fulfilling for patients and their loved ones. Attuned to the possibilities of sensory spirituality, we can enhance a peaceful, even joyful participation in the encounter with mystery that dying entails. In the process, we can learn something of our own spiritual journeys ourselves.

The problem of integrating relevant spiritual care may be one of place and method, not of inclination or intent. Attention must be paid to how people know, so that strategies for intervention will be appropriate. But there are rich resources which can serve as a starting point for more holistic interventions which are easily appropriated and adapted for providing spiritual care (Achterberg, Dossey, and Kolkmeier, 1994; Bailey, 1994). Most people are immensely grateful for the opportunity to enter into relationship and healing with their whole selves, and their creative experiences. By so doing, spirituality that is seeking the Wholly Other, experiencing the holy not just with the mind but with the whole body, can be facilitated. We can experience embodiment as sensory spirituality, and by so doing, encourage those for whom we care to join us on the journey–bodies, minds, spirits–and we become one with another–and with the One.

REFERENCES

Achterberg, J., Dossey, B., & Kolkmeier, L. (1994). *Rituals of healing: Using imagery for health and wellness.* New York: Bantam Books.

Astin, J.A. (1998). Why patients use alternative medicine: Results of a national study. *Journal of the American Medical Association* 279(19), 1548-1553.

Babler, J. (1997). A comparison of spiritual care provided by hospice social workers, nurses, and spiritual care professionals. *The Hospice Journal* 12(4), 15-27.

Bailey, S. (1997). The arts in spiritual care. *Seminars in Oncology Nursing* 13(4), 242-247.

Bailey, S. (1994). Creativity and the close of life. In I. Corless, B. Germino, & M. pop culture, and the arts. In Inge Corless, Barbara Germino, & Mary Pittman (Eds.), *Dying, death, and bereavement: Theoretical perspectives and other ways of knowing* (pp. 317-326). Boston: Jones and Bartlett.

Beck, S. L. (1991). The therapeutic use of music for cancer-related pain. *Oncology Nursing Forum* 18 (8), 1327-1337.

Bertman, S. (1994). Past the smart of feeling: Some images of grief in literature, pop culture, and the arts. In Inge Corless, Barbara Germino, & Mary Pittman (Eds.), *Dying, death, and bereavement: Theoretical perspectives and other ways of knowing* (pp. 317-326). Boston: Jones and Bartlett.

Brown-Saltzman, K. (1997). Replenishing the spirit by meditative prayer and guided imagery. *Seminars in Oncology Nursing* 13(4):255-259.

Burton, L.A. (1998). The spiritual dimension of palliative care. *Seminars in Oncology Nursing* 14(2):121-128.

Campbell, J. (1968) *The hero with a thousand faces* (2nd ed.). Princeton: Princeton University Press.

Cerrato, P.L. (1998). Spirituality and healing. *RN* 61(2):49-50.

Chandler, E. (1993). Can post-traumatic stress disorder be prevented? *Accident and Emergency Nursing* 1, 87-91.

Colt, G. H. (1996, September). The healing revolution. *Life*, 34-50.

Cousineau, P. (1995). *Soul: An Archeology.* San Francisco: HarperCollins.

Derrickson, B.S. (1996). The spiritual work of the dying: A framework and case studies. *The Hospice Journal* 11(2):11-30.

Dossey, L. (1993). *Healing words: The power of prayer and the practice of medicine.* San Francisco: HarperCollins.

Dyson, J., Cobb, M., & Forman, D. (1997), The meaning of spirituality: A literature review. *Journal of Advanced Nursing* 26(6):1183-1188.

Eisenberg, D.M., Davis, R.B., Eltner, S.L., Appel, S., Wilkey, S., Van Rompay, M., & Kessler, R.C. (1998). Trends in alternative medicine use in the United States, 1990-1997. *Journal of the American Medical Association* 280(18): 1569-1575.

Eisenberg, D. M., Kessler, R. C., Foster, C., Norlock, F., Colkins, D., & Delbanco, T. (1993). Unconventional medicine in the United States: Prevalence, costs, and patterns of use. *New England Journal of Medicine*, 328, 246-252.

Emblen, J.D. (1992). Religion and spirituality defined according to current use in nursing literature. *Journal of Professional Nursing* 8(1), 41-47.

Fehring, R.J., Miller, J.F., & Shaw, C. (1997). Spiritual well-being, religiosity, hope, depression, and other mood states in elderly people coping with cancer. *Oncology Nursing Forum* 24(4), 663-71.

Fischer, K.R. (1995). *Autumn gospel: Women in the second half of life.* New York: Paulist Press.

Halstead, M.T. & Mickley, J.R. (1997). Attempting to fathom the unfathomable: Descriptive views of spirituality. *Seminars in Oncology Nursing* 13(4), 225-230.

Koenig, H. G. (1995). Use of acute hospital services and mortality among religious and non-religious copers with medical illness. *Journal of Religious Gerontology* 9 (3), 1-22.

Koenig, H.G., Cohen, H., Blazer, D., Pieper, C., Meador, K., Shelp, F., Goli, V. & DiPasquale, B. (1992). Religious coping and depression among elderly, hospital-ized, medically ill men. *American Journal of Psychiatry* 149 (12), 1693-1700.

Levin, J. S. (1996). How prayer heals: A theoretical model. *Alternative Therapies* 2 (1), 66-73.

Macrae, J. (1995). Nightengale's spiritual philosophy and its significance for modern nursing. Image. *Journal of Nursing Scholarship*, 27, 8-10.

Martsolf, D.S. (1997). Cultural aspects of spirituality in cancer care. *Seminars in Oncology Nursing* 13(4), 231-236.

Matthews, D.A., McCullough, M.E., Larson, D.B., Koenig, H.G., Swyers, J.P., & Milano, M.G. (1998). Religious commitment and health status: A review of the research and implications for family practice. *Archives of Family Medicine* 7(2):118-124.

McGrath, P. (1997). Putting spirituality on the agenda: Hospice research findings on the 'ignored' dimension. *The Hospice Journal* 12(4):1-14.

Millison, M.B. (1995). A review of the research on spiritual care and hospice. *The Hospice Journal* 10(4):3-18.

Mickley, J., Soeken, K., & Belcher, A. (1992). Spiritual well-being, religiousness, and hope among women with breast cancer. *Image: Journal of Nursing Scholar-ship*, 24, 267-272.

Moore, T. (1992). *Care of the soul: A guide for cultivating depth and sacredness in everyday life.* New York: HarperCollins.

Nelson, J. B. (1992). *Body theology.* Louisville: Westminster/John Knox Press.

Norris, K. (1993). *Dakota: A spiritual geography.* Boston: Houghton Mifflin.

Perlman, D. & Takacs, G. J. (1990). *The 10 stages of change.* Nursing Management 21 (4), 33-38.

Samuels, M. (1995). Art as a healing force. *Alternative Therapies,* 1, 38-40.

Schroeder-Sheker, T. (1994). Music for the dying: A personal account of the new field of music thanantology-history, theories, and clinical narratives. *Journal of Holistic Nursing,* 12, 83-99.

Simpkinson, C., & Simpkinson, A. (Eds.). (1993). *Sacred stories: A celebration of the power of stories to transform and heal.* San Francisco: HarperCollins.

Taylor, E.J. (1997). The story behind the story: The use of storytelling in spiritual caregiving. *Seminars in Oncology Nursing* 13(4):252-254.

Thompson, M. (1995). *Soul feast: An invitation to the Christian spiritual life.* Louisville: Westminster/John Knox Press.

Wallis, C. (1996). Faith and healing. *New York Times* 147 (26), 58-70.

Whitcomb, J.B. (1993). The way to go home: Creating comfort through therapeutic music and milieu. *The American Journal of Alzheimer's Care and Related Disorders & Research* 6, 1-10.

Access to Care

Constance M. Dahlin

SUMMARY. In the twenty years since the National Hospice Organization began, hospice has grown tremendously. However, it still only serves a small percentage of terminally ill patients. This is because access to hospice services is limited by various restrictions to care. These barriers to care include societal attitudes towards death, diversity issues, socioeconomic issues, and eligibility issues. In order to develop and serve more of the population, hospice agencies must be flexible, creative, and use ingenuity to bridge the gaps that occur for some terminally ill patients. *[Article copies available for a fee from The Haworth Document Delivery Service: 1-800-342-9678. E-mail address: getinfo@haworthpressinc.com <Website: http://www.haworthpressinc.com>]*

KEYWORDS. Hospice, access, criteria

INTRODUCTION

As the National Hospice Organization enters its 20th year, hospice in America has certainly grown. There are currently some 3,000 hospices across the country serving approximately 450,000 dying persons.[1] Within the 10 years I have been a hospice and palliative care nurse, hospice has been defined by the Medicare benefit, with most hospices being Medicare certified and receiving payment for services. In addition, in the late '80s, hospice was working hard to establish itself and to promote more public discussions about death and dying. Now, end-of-life care is currently a popular and well-publicized topic. However, from my perspective, hospice in America is not fully woven

---

[Haworth co-indexing entry note]: "Access to Care." Dahlin, Constance M. Co-published simultaneously in *The Hospice Journal* (The Haworth Press, Inc.) Vol. 14, No. 3/4, 1999, pp. 75-84; and: *The Hospice Heritage: Celebrating Our Future* (ed: Inge B. Corless and Zelda Foster) The Haworth Press, Inc., 1999, pp. 75-84. Single or multiple copies of this article are available for a fee from The Haworth Document Delivery Service [1-800-342-9678, 9:00 a.m. - 5:00 p.m. (EST). E-mail address: getinfo@haworthpressinc.com].

into the fabric of care at the end of life. Working in the hospital as a palliative care nurse practitioner, I see many people who are unable to receive hospice care because of various impediments blocking access to hospice services. These barriers limit the optimal supportive care measures necessary to promote a "good death" at home and prevent appropriate bereavement follow-up to cope with death.

Statistics show that annually only 15-20% of people die within hospice.[2] Another 65-80% of patients die in an inpatient setting with approximately 15% of those deaths occurring in long term care settings. Of the 15-20% of patients served by hospice, the majority are white adults.[3] Minorities are not well represented in these statistics. However, access is not merely a racial issue. From my own work experiences within an East Coast urban hospice serving the inner city as well as in a West Coast smaller and more rural hospice, access is influenced by other varied factors including societal attitudes regarding death, diversity issues, economic issues, and admission criteria.

SOCIETAL PERSPECTIVE OF DEATH

In the United States, there have been a multitude of technological advances in health care. Patients have more treatment possibilities than ever before, as there are myriad treatments or procedures offered to patients. Therefore, treatment for life threatening diseases continues much longer. The question is what difference a given treatment or procedure will make to the patient's outcome; more specifically the benefit and the burden of the treatment or procedure itself. For some people, stopping such treatments can be seen as giving up on a patient or forgoing hope. Likewise, forgoing treatment, withdrawing treatment, or stopping treatment is often perceived as hastening death. After all, within the medical community, death is still often viewed as failure, rather than the inevitable process of a person with advanced, life threatening illness or the relief of the person who is suffering. Changing this perspective through education initiatives is in various stages within medicine, nursing, and other allied health professions.[4]

Since hospice philosophy espouses stopping aggressive treatments, many patients and health care clinicians perceive hospice as death. Thus, many patients are denied hospice services because a physician may find it difficult to stop life prolonging treatments at all costs, or patients may not agree to cessation of these procedures. In such situations, quality of life looms in the background but is never brought to the foreground for discussion.

Additionally, many patients do not realize that they have the right to refuse treatment or that the hospice option is even available when they have decided to stop "fighting the good fight." Moreover, although hospice is well known to clinicians caring for patients at the end of their lives, hospice is still not an entity well-known to the public. Hospice care remains an infrequently discussed topic. Circumstances may necessitate it. To this end, many states have begun initiatives whose goal is to improve care at the end-of-life through both professional and public education.

DIVERSITY ISSUES

Race

As previously stated, hospice tends to serve a mostly white middle-class population.[4] This Caucasian population has enjoyed a high standard of hospital care without fear of discrimination or recrimination. For non-Caucasians, however, health care has not necessarily been equal or without prejudice.[5] Some cultural minorities may want to be assured that every possible treatment or procedure is being done. Otherwise, the result is feelings of uncertainty as to why treatments may be withheld or withdrawn and feelings of discrimination that the underlying reason for this occurrence might be to save money and technology for other individuals. Therefore, not initiating treatment or withdrawal of treatment is a delicate situation to minorities who feel they do not receive the same standard of healthcare. The result is mistrust about care at the end of life.[5]

Understandably, to minorities, the hospice philosophy may be perceived as giving up and not pursuing possible care options. Few hospices have done outreach to change such perceptions of care nor are there many hospices reaching out to care for culturally diverse populations. Indeed, many agencies are not serving inner city areas where race may influence acceptance of hospice service.

Culture

Another factor influencing access to hospice services is culture. Many hospices neither have minority representation on their staff nor have the resources readily available to appropriately provide care for culturally diverse individuals. This lack of diversity is particularly reflected when observing the attendance at various hospice conferences. Therefore, it is difficult to justify making hospice referrals to individuals of diverse cultures, knowing there will be language barriers or lack of knowledge about cultural or religious beliefs. This is especially true when individuals might be better served by a home care agency that hires multi-cultural staff. For instance, there is a large Chinese community in the city where I work. Within that community, there is a home care agency with bilingual staff. This ability to feel understood both in translation of healthcare needs, health care practices, and cultural rituals, may be more important to a patient and family than the possible benefits of hospice.

Moreover, hospice most often views the death process from the western European-American perspective. That is, the patient is the focus of care, informed of the disease process, and is personally responsible for making decisions about her or his care. However, this perspective can cause problems in some eastern cultures where health care issues are not discussed with an individual patient, and instead, the family is responsible for decision-making,

When a patient speaks a foreign language, further problems may ensue. It is my experience that most hospices are not adequately equipped to deal with clients speaking languages other than English. This is demonstrated by admission and election forms that patient and family must sign that are usually only in English. In my years in hospice, I cannot recall ever having seen or worked on translations of admitting forms other than Spanish. More distressing is that many hospice personnel do not know about resources such as the AT&T Language Line Services to enable optimal translation and respect of various cultures.

Thus, without cultural sensitivity and knowledge of cultural elements other than Caucasian, culturally diverse patients will not elect hospice. In these cases, cultural minorities may only be cared for by family members instead of professionals.

Religious Diversity

Historically, hospice has its foundations in the Christian tradition. Indeed, some names of hospices are very Christian such as Good Samaritan, or Sacred Heart. These undertones can cause discomfort for people of Non-Christian faiths such as Jews, Muslims, and Native Americans who may perceive little sensitivity to their own rituals or they may feel that there may be covert attempts to convert them to Christian religions. Moreover, since religion is linked to culture, discussion in regards to decision-making surrounding health care treatments, the meaning of pain as well as the meaning of death, may be additionally difficult. There may not be a common language or the understanding of religious principles among hospice workers to discuss these sensitive issues. For instance, Jehovah's Witnesses may not want blood treatments for leukemia, Cambodians may refuse surgery for colon disturbance, and Jews have particular burial needs.[6] Furthermore, providing spiritual support may be biased. Whereas in western traditions organized prayer may be common, eastern traditions may practice frequent meditation. Thus the lack of understanding about these religious traditions means a less that satisfying experience within hospice, and can actually alienate the patient and family from hospice workers. Hospice providers need to understand a wide range of religious founding principles and integrate them into a unique care plan.

In addition, the issue of bereavement follow-up is very much directed to the Christian tradition and English speaking individuals. Again, there may not be personnel who can appropriately discuss the death experience and its meaning within a diverse culture. Grief reactions may be misinterpreted or overlooked.[6] Additionally, there may be lack of translators to understand the subtleties of coping with death.

ECONOMICS

Insurance

Medicare is the largest payor for hospice, covering approximately 65% of hospice patients.[4] In addition, 43 state Medicaid programs cover hospice. However, for younger patients who have commercial insurance, a hospice benefit may not be part of their insurance package. Insurance case managers may lack understanding as to what defines hospice services. The result is that insurance companies may piece together elements of terminal care that lack the integrated, holistic approach of hospice care. Unfortunately under this circumstance, a patient and family forgo the comprehensive, interdisciplinary expertise and support provided by hospice during the dying process.

Patients without any insurance usually lose out completely. Though most hospices say they will serve patients regardless of ability to pay, the reality is more complicated. These days, in my experience, fewer hospice agencies provide free care.[4] If an agency does, it may only allow one free care patient to be on the census at a time. Even so, the care is different. In my experience, when free care is provided, it is usually limited to specific disciplines. Most commonly included are nursing and home health aide services and possibly volunteers. In addition, there may be limited medications and fewer visits. Thus patients without insurance usually cannot access full hospice services. Yet, such patients can benefit the most from hospice since they may have the least supports in place.

Geography

Geography can greatly influence access to care.[7] Usually it is lower socioeconomic areas such as rural poor or city poor that lack services. In large states such as Oregon, Washington, Texas, or Colorado, there can be lack of services in wilderness areas or rural areas. Paradoxically, services are often unavailable in large inner cities or slums such as in cities such as Boston, New York, Detroit, or Chicago. In inner cities, safety and acceptance limit the round the clock availability of services.[7] Patients and families may relocate to relatives' houses in suburban areas to qualify for services. In rural areas, the large geographic distances may prohibit the intensive and supportive services hospice can provide. Indeed, patients and families may move to a larger town or area to receive health care services.

HOSPICE ADMISSION CRITERIA

Prognosis

Estimating terminal prognosis is a major barrier to hospice care.[7] Many physicians are intimidated by making a 6-month prognosis. This is true particularly since the onset of Operation Restore Trust. The myth persists that if the patient lives longer than expected, Medicare will somehow punish the referring physician. What many physicians do not realize is that certifying a terminal illness is done according to "the best of their knowledge." Moreover, hospice agencies review patient cases every 3 months to make sure patients still fit the terminal criteria. However, many physicians feel it is easier to give prognoses for cancer diagnoses rather than non-cancer diagnoses. Thus, hospice, to a large extent, still cares primarily for cancer patients upon whom the tenets of hospice care were built. Non-cancer diagnoses such as heart disease, pulmonary disease, neurological diseases, and AIDS are difficult to predict in terms of their course. Because hospice was modeled around terminal oncology care, patients living with non-cancer diseases have not been well integrated into hospice care. The result is many terminally ill patients are not offered the hospice option.

Eligibility

Looking at the Medicare guidelines, eligibility is defined as having Medicare Part A insurance benefits in addition to having a terminal illness.[8] However, in reality, eligibility criteria varies by hospice agency. Eligibility requirements include the presence of a primary caregiver, whether or not to accept patients with tube feedings or IVs or persons with non-cancer diagnoses. The lack of uniformity regarding types of treatments received by potential hospice patients that are acceptable to hospice agencies, confuses the specific defining criteria for hospice. Non-hospice clinicians do not understand that each hospice agency may have its own criteria for admission, but that these are more specific and financially based that what is defined in the Medicare regulations. Instead, the inclination is to take that one hospice's admission criteria and generalize it to all hospices, leading to more misperceptions of hospice philosophy and care. The major variations of admission criteria include the necessity of a primary caregiver, acceptable treatments, and patient location.

The first criterion is the presence of a primary caregiver. Although it is not in the Medicare regulations, many hospices demand a primary caregiver.[8] This is usually defended by the professional management clause that states a hospice must ensure that services are provided in a safe and effective manner with little risk. Some hospice agencies are fairly lenient with defining safe care and maintain the spirit of hospice care within any setting. Other hospice agencies interpret Medicare regulations to the "letter of the law." This strict interpretation excludes patients who have no family, or no family willing and able to take on the burdens of care. In many families, both heads of household must work to support the family, which leaves no one to assume domestic duties. In other circumstances, patients have been "loners" all their lives and do not want or do not have extended friends or relatives who can assist in end-of-life care. In addition, many patients may have a debilitated family member who is physically with the patient but is not able to do much care. Furthermore, there are homeless people and people with mental illnesses that live in settings they call home, but which are not quite the "safe" home that hospices deem appropriate. However, many of these patients could be safely cared for within the setting they call "home" until they decline. Arrangements can be made and events anticipated so that the patient is allowed to stay in the comfort of those surroundings if they so chose.

The second criterion is the type of treatments hospice may accept. Hospice agencies vary widely with regard to what are considered curative versus palliative treatments. Although, it is not in the Medicare regulations, some programs demand a Do Not Resuscitate (DNR) order while others do not. Some will accept feeding tubes or hydration and others will not. Some will let patients utilize oral antibiotics or others will not. Consequently, there is inconsistency in what is defined as hospice care which is confusing for many clinicians, let alone the general public. The result is professional frustration regarding the lack of uniform admissions criteria and an ensuing reluctance to refer to hospice. Thus, patients continue to receive their care from the model of acute care without the benefit of coordinated, comprehensive care at home.

The third criterion is location of patient. There are many patients with underlying mental illness or developmental delays who develop a terminal illness. These include patients with mental illnesses, genetic illnesses, addiction disorders, and personality disorders. This special population may live in group homes, halfway houses, or mental institutions. These patients lack good access to routine medical care, let alone access to the specialized services needed for the care of person with a terminal illness. With the onset of an incurable disease, the patients may experience beneficent neglect and not be referred to any agencies that could offer assistance.

However, concomitant with the lack of basic medical care which would help direct care are marginal living conditions that act as barriers to receiving hospice care. For both the frail elderly and the mentally ill, the individual patient's housing situation may restrict care. In some facilities, there may be inadequate personnel to administer care to the patient when she or he is declining. Furthermore, there may be inconsistent caregivers since health care workers may rotate. Similarly, there may be inadequate caregivers. Other clients residing in the house who might serve as informal caregivers may also have mental illnesses and infirmities that diminish their ability to assist in caring for the patient. Additionally, there is the concern of informed consent for a client if she or he is not able to understand the nature of his or her illness. Most frustrating and time consuming are dealing with the usual bureaucracy that surrounds these settings. At the core of this issue, however, is the lack of education for hospice caregivers to deal with patients with pre-existing mental illnesses. The result is that many mentally ill patients who develop terminal illnesses lack the attention to and the benefit of the expert pain and symptom management hospice could provide.

CONCLUSION

Since hospice care is utilized by only a small percentage of dying patients, access may ultimately affect the long-term success or failure of hospice as it is known today. With the focus on end-of-life care, and the integration of hospice into the specialty of palliative medicine, hospices agencies must demonstrate their flexibility and ingenuity to assist in removing barriers to care. First and foremost, hospice organizations need to reevaluate their mission and goals. There needs to be the commitment to seek out underserved populations. In particular, this includes the development of more multifaceted cultural training and education within hospice agencies, themselves, to develop cultural competence.[9] Simultaneously, hospice agencies need to reach out to diverse communities to create liaison relationships and employ community members.

Second, with the changes in Medicare covering both home care and hospice, it is doubtful that hospice lengths of stay will increase. Indeed, everyone in the health care industry states that patients are more acutely ill and inpatient stays are increasing.[7] Patients and caregivers are caught in a bind. Some patients are neither sick, nor able to care for themselves at home, nor terminally ill enough for hospice. The result is forgoing any services at all and experiencing multiple, sequential hospitalizations. Thus, the ongoing re-evaluation of the effectiveness of the Medicare benefit is critical in order to revise the benefit to incorporate current technology. In addition, there needs to be Federal legislation to make hospice a universal component of all health insurance programs. Only then will more patients have appropriate access; access that is not dictated by the type of insurance plan. In the meantime, pre-hospice and bridge programs will gain popularity because patients can still receive terminal care with support even if they do not qualify for or are not appropriate for hospice.

Finally, in order to improve access to care, there must be more flexibility and creativity on the part of hospice agencies. Caring for underserved populations and culturally diverse populations is not easy. Some hospices may feel that it is too much of a burden to increase access to care. Building bridges takes time to plan interventions, energy to create working solutions, patience to work with resistant staff, and resources to acquire financial support for community initiatives. The overall result would be not only an improvement of quality of life for increasing numbers of terminally ill patients, but also improvement of the overall quality of care to the terminally ill population as a whole. To me this is most important and will ensure the viability of hospice in the future.

REFERENCES

1. National Hospice Organization. (1997). *National Hospice Census.*

2. Cassel, C.K.; Vladek, B.C. (1996). Sounding Board-ICD9 Code for Palliative or Terminal Care. *N Engl J Med* 355:1232.

3. Christakis N.A.; Escarce, J.J. (1996). Survival of Medicare Patients after Enrollment in Hospice Programs. *N Engl J Med.* 335:172-178.

4. Merritt, D.; Fox-Grange, W.; Rothouse, M.; Lynn, L.; Cohn, F.; Forlini, J.H. (1998). *State Initiatives in End-of-Life Care–Policy Guide for State Legislators.* Washington, DC: National Conference of State Legislators.

5. Krakauer, E.L. (1997). Commentary on Mistrust Racism, and End-of-Life Treatment. *Hastings Center Report.* May-June:23-24.

6. Kirkwood, N.A. (1993) *A Hospital Handbook in Multiculturalism and Religion.* Alexandria, Australia: Millennium Books.

7. National Hospice Organization. (1998). *Committee on the Medicare Hospice Benefit & End-of-Life Care.*

8. U.S. Dept of Health and Human Services, Health Care Financing Administration. (1983). *Medicare Program; Hospice Care; Final Rule.* Friday December 16, Federal Register. 48: 243.

9. Lipson, J.G. (1996). *Culturally Competent Care in Culture and Nursing Care–A Pocket Guide.* San Francisco: UCSF Nursing Press.

End of Life Care and Decision Making:
How Far We Have Come,
How Far We Have to Go

Connie Zuckerman
David Wollner

SUMMARY. While enormous progress has been made in improving the quality of care and the decision-making process for patients at the end of life, as a society we still have far to go to ensure that dying patients and their families have a comfortable and dignified death. In particular, reexamination and reconfiguration of our current decision framework is essential as our elderly population with chronic disease and slowly fatal conditions expands. With less certain disease paths and more complex and ambiguous choices, the growth of this geriatric population challenges us to develop a broader conceptualization of end of life care planning, so that end of life considerations are integrated into a larger anticipatory framework addressing options and needs as patients gradually decline. Within this framework hospice becomes a natural, integrated option along a continuum of care planning, rather than an abrupt alternative at a late stage of illness. End of life care planning must positively anticipate a robust array of needs and concerns well beyond the dramatic decisions to withhold or withdraw life-prolonging technologies usually found in advance directives. To embrace this broader framework it is critical that primary care physicians as well as disease specialists receive training in fundamental aspects of both geriatric and palliative care. Professionals from both of these disciplines must share expertise with each other, and should collaborate in advocacy efforts to effectuate changes in the clinical, policy and legislative

[Haworth co-indexing entry note]: "End of Life Care and Decision Making: How Far We Have Come, How Far We Have to Go." Zuckerman, Connie, and David Wollner. Co-published simultaneously in *The Hospice Journal* (The Haworth Press, Inc.) Vol. 14, No. 3/4, 1999, pp. 85-107; and: *The Hospice Heritage: Celebrating Our Future* (ed: Inge B. Corless and Zelda Foster) The Haworth Press, Inc., 1999, pp. 85-107. Single or multiple copies of this article are available for a fee from The Haworth Document Delivery Service [1-800-342-9678, 9:00 a.m. - 5:00 p.m. (EST). E-mail address: getinfo@haworthpressinc. com].

arenas. *[Article copies available for a fee from The Haworth Document Delivery Service: 1-800-342-9678. E-mail address: getinfo@haworthpressinc.com <Website: http://www.haworthpressinc.com>]*

KEYWORDS. Palliative care, geriatric care, advance care planning, end of life care

INTRODUCTION

Rose K., an 84 year old widow, was a weary veteran in the war against death. Her husband had died six years earlier during surgery for a leaky heart valve. One of her daughters had died just two years ago, suffering from lung cancer. Although currently healthy, Rose could envision her own future. She declared to her remaining daughters, "I don't ever want to suffer like your dear sister." Active in her synagogue, Rose appointed her Rabbi as her health care proxy. She instructed him, "I want to live every minute I can, but not a second longer than I must."

A short time later, Rose collapsed while shopping. Complete heart block and heart failure were diagnosed. With proper care and rehabilitation, Rose returned home four weeks later, assisted by a visiting nurse and a home health aide. Although deeply concerned, her remaining two daughters were largely uninvolved in her care, as they were busy with their own careers and families. But Rose was content–she didn't want to burden them anyway.

Rose's new physician, a cardiologist, proclaimed that with her new pacemaker and medications, she was "out of the woods." Rose's entreaties to discuss advance directives with him were rebuffed: "You could live another ten years!" her cardiologist replied.

During the next year, Rose began to decline. Chest pains, fatigue, nightly breathlessness all began to creep into her daily life. After consulting her Rabbi, Rose asked her cardiologist to issue a DNR order for her. He was reluctant, but eventually relented.

Over the next five months, Rose was hospitalized three times for refractory heart failure. Her chest pain continued unabated, and upon her eventual return home she required 24 hour care. She became listless and ate little. Finally, through the persistence of her Rabbi, Rose was once again brought to the hospital. Her two daughters were summoned, each carrying the weight of her own fears about Rose. One daughter, Miriam, demanded everything be done for her mother, and gladly signed the consent forms for the suggested cardiac surgery. The other, Rachel, grieving at her mother's suffering, just wanted to "end it all." The Rabbi also arrived, making clear that Rose never wanted any type of heart surgery.

While they debated what to do for Rose, her condition deteriorated. She moaned in pain. She became incontinent and agitated. The cardiologist grew adamant that Rose would die without the surgery, his opinion having been confirmed by several colleagues. Miriam agreed, yet Rachel asked that her mother just be given morphine for her pain. Upon hearing the Rabbi's suggestion that perhaps a hospice referral was appropriate, the cardiologist responded that hospice was for terminal cancer patients.

That evening, as the cardiologist left the hospital, he suggested they all reconvene in the morning to re-evaluate Rose's condition. The Rabbi was told that he, too, had to leave the hospital, as visiting hours had ended. Sometime that evening Rose died, though because she was alone, the time of her death was not clearly known.

Over the past several decades, a remarkable and evolving dialogue has emerged in this country concerning the care that patients receive at the end of their lives. Among professional organizations, in the public arena, and even in the privacy of individual homes, interest in death and the process of dying has taken hold. The questions that have surfaced, and the answers that have evolved in response, have addressed a range of matters, from the pragmatic to the most profound: How are we likely to die? What are our goals for care at the end of life? Who ought to be involved in decisions about such care? What are the critical decisions that need to be made when a patient is facing death? Where is the best setting for patients to die? At home? In the hospital? In some other type of health care facility? When is the ideal time for end of life discussions to begin? And finally, and perhaps most difficult to answer, why, after all the progress that has been made, do we still encounter tragedies such as that experienced by Rose and her family, and how can we do better for such patients? Some of these questions have generated thoughtful responses and genuine improvements in clinical settings and in the public domain. In private settings, many families, friends, patients and their providers have worked together to construct care plans that are respectful of individual values and that ensure a comfortable and dignified death. But all too often, as reflected in the true story of Rose, reality falls far short of the ideal, and patients and their loved ones suffer terribly as a result.

In many respects, as a society we have made enormous progress, given that discussion of death and dying has only recently emerged as appropriate and acceptable. Some, including far too many clinicians, still find it difficult and troubling to raise and anticipate the specter of death. But many notable, indeed remarkable, accomplishments have been achieved over the last several decades: The central role of the patient's values and choices in decisions about end of life care is firmly rooted in the legal pronouncements and ethical analyses that frame our discussions about death and dying. Legal mechanisms have been constructed to help stimulate and guide discussions, and to facilitate an orderly decision making process when patients can no longer speak for themselves. Thousands of patients and their grateful families have benefited from the compassion and care provided by hospice programs. Exciting initiatives and programs have been launched to test new ideas, to generate useful data, and to enhance access to hospice and palliative care for all dying patients, no matter what their struggles or circumstances. Yet Rose died alone and in pain. How far have we really come and how far do we yet have to go?

Rose had strong lucid opinions about her preferences and priorities as her life began to draw to a close. She had taken the recommended step of appointing a health care proxy and articulating her wishes. She began to consider her choices well before the moment of crisis. She had taken the initiative to have a Do Not Resuscitate order issued in advance. She had been logical and thoughtful, not shying away from some of the difficult decisions that faced her. Yet as her health began to fail, and her condition deteriorated, her story began to look all too familiar: ambiguity, conflicting goals, uncertainty and emotional turmoil all took center stage, eclipsing Rose's previous pronouncements and relegating her proxy to a marginal role. Her wishes, to the extent they were known, were never fully considered nor integrated into the plan of care. Her daughters, while not formally appointed surrogates, clearly saw a role for themselves, as intimates who were deeply touched by her dying. They were left conflicted, guilt ridden and in crisis. Her hospice referral, such as it was, was rebuffed by a misinformed physician, and came far too late to be of value to Rose or her family. In many ways, the circumstances surrounding her death were unnecessary and tragic–and an all too common occurrence, even in today's more enlightened environment. Unfortunately, Rose's death reflected not an anomaly, but more the norm–a very troubling norm given the enormous size of our aging population, our increasingly multicultural society, and our expanding array of treatment options that potentially prolong life.

END OF LIFE CARE FOR WHOM?
AN EVOLVING PATIENT PROFILE

If demographic trends continue along their current path, patients such as Rose will increasingly come to dominate our focus and discussions concerning end of life care. In many ways decisionally capable patients with a predictable disease course, such as cancer patients, have helped us understand our obligations for pain control, symptom management, and other essential aspects of hospice and palliative care. Young victims of accidents and trauma have helped propel death and dying into the judicial and policy arenas. It will increasingly, however, be elderly patients with chronic diseases and diminished functional capacity who push us to reconsider our current end of life care and decision framework. Elderly patients with "slowly fatal conditions," as Joanne Lynn has so astutely described them (Lynn, 1997), constitute the fastest growing segment of our population. Accompanying this growth are enormously complex medical and social phenomena that defy simple categorization or simplistic mechanisms for addressing end of life decisions.

The explosion of our elderly population, particularly of individuals 85 and older, reflects both tremendous success in public health and medical management, and enormous complexity, as we grapple with medical and social situations which our current systems of care delivery were never designed to address. By the year 2030 fully 20% of our population will be over the age of 65 (Institute of Medicine, 1997). This will begin to emerge as a significant cumulative growth of disability and chronic illness. While there is no doubt that strategies of "successful aging" will enable more and more individuals to live longer lives of better quality, it is also inevitable that as we age as a society, we will begin to witness the increasing incidence of those conditions and diseases which plague the elderly in acute, chronic and ultimately fatal ways. Sixty percent of all cancer-associated deaths in this country occur in individuals over 65 (Cleary & Carbone, 1997), yet these deaths account for only 23% of the deaths in our elderly patient population (Cassel & Siegel, 1998). The majority of elderly individuals instead become afflicted with, and *eventually* die from, diseases and complications such as stroke, heart disease, dementia, pneumonia, and respiratory and multi-organ failure (Institute of Medicine 1997). What stands out so starkly is that these are all medical conditions that are at the heart of geriatric medicine, yet that lie outside of the traditional disease courses associated with hospice care.

The progression from chronic, debilitating illness to an eventually terminal condition is characterized by unpredictability: Through a mix of proactive steps, aggressive medical management and monitoring, and other unknown factors, patients with slowly fatal conditions may live years in circumstances that diminish their once youthful capacity yet do not deposit them on death's doorstep. There may be periods of relative stability marked by occasional acute crises. There may be gradual diminution in physical and functional capacity, and increasing dependence on relatives and paid caregivers. Incremental physical losses and social isolation may characterize their day to day lives, and their cognitive abilities may gradually decline as a result or in consort. Yet certain medical interventions may ameliorate these symptoms or even restore functioning in circumstances previously considered inevitable aspects of the aging process. In fact, geriatric practitioners increasingly look at many symptoms and conditions as remediable and reversible, rather than merely accepting them as a consequence of old age. How, then, does one begin to confront issues of end of life in patients who may justifiably look to medical progress and new innovations as their welcome companions rather than as their adversaries?

Into this mix of slowly progressive illness and gradual functional decline is often an ever expanding role for "informal" caregivers, usually family members or other intimate loved ones whose caregiving participation is the cement that bonds the care plan together. The role of such family members is frequently much more complex and intertwined with the patient's interests than our usual "autonomy" decision framework concedes (Levine and Zuckerman, 1999). Patient self-determination remains the core foundation upon which care decisions should be built. However, simplistic notions of patient autonomy may ring hollow when clinical care plans rely upon the intense physical and emotional involvement of intimate loved ones. Family members often play a critical role, as direct caregivers, as negotiators of care systems, and at times as surrogate decision makers. Particularly in this climate of outpatient, home-based care, family can be assigned essential caregiving responsibilities far beyond the surrogate decision role, without ever receiving sufficient information, support or ongoing training. Hospice is the only care framework that explicitly acknowledges a more complex presence for the family, recognizing that patients are usually part of a broader "unit" of care and acknowledging the needs and interests of other members of the unit. However, even hospice benefits, in their current configuration, anticipate enormous caregiving contributions from involved loved ones. Even the most selfless of caregivers may find this challenging, especially if they have already spent years caring for a relative with a slowly fatal condition.

Finally, along with this expanding geriatric patient population comes the increasing incidence of dementia and diminished cognitive abilities. While many elderly patients are fully capable of articulating their needs and their medical problems, an increasing number will gradually lose that ability. Thus their subjective experiences and the symptoms that plague them may slip from sight and sound and become undetectable to involved clinicians. While in a few select cases an advance directive can address some of these concerns, the reality is that most advance directives do not address the less dramatic but equally important issues, both medical and social, that arise in the day to day living that precedes dying. Furthermore, no advance directive can adequately unmask the pain or other symptoms that demented patients may experience but that are hidden from detection because the patient can no longer speak for herself (Sengstaken & King, 1993). The loss of one's voice has profound impact, not only on the process of dying but on the day to day caregiving that precedes it, when quality palliative care could add such value to life. Thus arises the need to anticipate and perhaps assume the presence of certain symptoms, even in the absence of their acknowledged existence, in order to ensure adequate symptom management for such patients. Working with an increasing number of demented elderly will mean our clinical skills to detect and anticipate pain and other symptoms will need to be all the more sharp and focused. This will not be easy, given how poorly we currently manage the symptoms and pain of late stage illness even in patients who can speak for themselves.

The picture that emerges, then, is of a complex patient population, with no one definitive path nor timetable toward death, who may ambivalently, at best, acknowledge and accept the emerging end of their lives. They may not possess the emboldened autonomy that our decision models uphold as desirable in formulating end of life care plans. They may lack the capacity to express the most fundamental and basic requests for pain alleviation and, even if eligible, they may not have the cognitive ability to request hospice care. We have paid little attention to this set of circumstances that all too frequently precedes the very end of life, as though we can cleanly excise the "terminal stage" from all that preceded it. What may be necessary in response, then, is a genuine reconsideration and reconfiguration of our current systems for addressing end of life care, and for training clinicians to be at their best in caring for patients who slowly progress toward the inevitable end of life.

CURRENT DECISION MAKING FRAMEWORKS: ARE THE INTERESTS OF PATIENTS ADVANCED BY ADVANCE DIRECTIVES?

In many ways, Rose was unusual in her advance consideration of death and dying. Only a small percentage of patients execute such directives in advance of incapacity (Lynn & Teno, 1993). Prompted by the experiences endured by her loved ones, Rose was able to reflect upon and express her own wishes concerning some of the more dramatic choices that might arise as life drew to a close: Her health care proxy was in place, a DNR order was on her chart, and she had articulated a philosophy that suggested that quality of life, rather than length of life, was most important to her. Only a small minority of patients have the ability or foresight to consider such concerns in advance. According to current models of end of life decision making, Rose had taken all the right steps to help ensure that her autonomous wishes would be respected. Yet ultimately this advance planning did not lead to a peaceful, dignified death for Rose, an all too common fate for patients in such circumstances.

As we have increasingly learned over the years, would that it were so simple. Through our collective clinical experiences and through research studies examining communication, advance care planning, surrogate decision making and other aspects of end of life care, we now know that the simple and elegant notion of patient autonomy is enormously challenging to implement in clinical reality, no matter how well intentioned we are. For patients with decisional capacity and clear, articulated choices, inadequate clinical training and a host of other organizational and professional barriers often frustrate desired plans and a dignified death (Institute of Medicine, 1997). For patients who lose decisional capacity, health care proxies, livings wills, and other advance planning mechanisms have all been promoted as important tools to foster frank and open communication about end of life care and to promote more patient-centered care decision making. Enormous resources have been spent promoting the use and integration of advance directives into the health care arena. Federal legislation known as the Patient Self-Determination Act requires health care providers to inform patients of the existence and availability of such mechanisms (Omnibus Budget Reconciliation Act, 1990). Numerous quantitative and qualitative studies have attempted to determine whether and how these mechanisms can truly promote and facilitate the type of decision making held up to be the ideal (Fischer, Tulsky, Rose et al., 1998; Teno, Licks, Lynn et al., 1997). While no conclusions can be definitively drawn, it is clear that all of these mechanisms have their flaws, and none have been enthusiastically embraced by the majority of patients for whom they are intended.

Health care agents, while of potential value (particularly in clarifying the legal authority of a surrogate decision maker) often lack the training, support or the strength to boldly assert the patient's choices and values (Dubler, 1995). They are sometimes unaware of the appointment itself, and even if aware, have not usually had the robust discussions necessary to undergird their role as the patient's designated spokesperson and surrogate decision maker. Even in situations where it appears conversations took place, their role may be thwarted or diminished, as was the case with Rose's Rabbi. Either formerly appointed, or informally stepping into place, it is also difficult for such surrogates to disentangle themselves from their own feelings and emotions about the situation. There is growing empirical evidence that the wishes they express on behalf of patients frequently do not match actual choices articulated by such patients (Suhl, Simons, Reedy & Garrick, 1994; Hare, Pratt & Nelson 1992). Whether or not this arrangement actually promotes patient autonomy in the usual clinical situation, therefore, is questionable.

For intimate loved ones, the end of life is rarely a time for cool reflection and disengaged consideration of a logical course of care, even if the patient did previously articulate clear wishes. Rose's daughter Miriam reflected the very intricate array of emotion, guilt and confusion that family members often feel as the reality of their loved one's approaching death grows clearer. Jumping at one more chance or clinging to one more opportunity may not seem irrational or illogical, particularly if the family has accompanied the patient on previous roller coaster rides through chronic illness and decline. It's easy to know in hindsight that the end of life has arrived–it's much harder to predict it going forward. And, as Rachel and Miriam so vividly demonstrated, it's not uncommon for family members to possess conflicting attitudes, each of them having some legitimacy if examined in the context of the broader scope of previous family relationships. The elegant notion of autonomous decision making, devoid of the complications that normally envelope intimate relationships and acute crises, may be an oversimplified way to approach such care decisions. Yet this is the model to which we are anchored.

Advance directives, and the broader notion of advance care planning, try to capture and reign in the complexity of such decisions by allowing us to anticipate and consider choices in advance of incapacity and the chaos brought on by acute crisis. In the typical use of an advance directive, distinct decision points are plucked from the course of continuing clinical care and elevated for careful advance scrutiny. Usually, a series of "rejections" are set up for the patient to select: I *do not* want CPR; I *do not* want to be connected to a ventilator; I *do not* want artificial nutrition and hydration; I *do not* want to go on living if I can no longer recognize my loved ones. It is, by and large, a profoundly sad reflection of what *not* to do for patients such as Rose, rather than an exploration of how best to support such patients as their conditions eventually become fatal.

Not all, but most patients who utilize advance directives are guided by this scenario. While such directives are theoretically available for individuals no matter what their care choices or concerns, the reality is that they are usually associated with withholding or withdrawing life-sustaining care. Such a course of action is then often linked with legitimate patient fears of abandonment or disquieting words from clinicians about "nothing more to be done." Perhaps this was the right decision framework for an earlier time when the excesses of paternalism were rampant in the clinical arena and access to quality hospice and palliative care was virtually non-existent. But at this time it is a decisional framework that reflects a poverty of vision about what *can* and ought to be done to *support* patients such as Rose who have ultimately fatal conditions. It projects a stagnant, snapshot image of the end of life, in contrast to the kinetics of change and uncertainty that often envelope end of life care and decision making. It is a simplistic framework at a time when choices are enormously complex and often ambiguous. For example, at least in some surveys, a significant proportion of older patients suggest they would not uniformly want to reject such treatment options (Cicirelli, 1997). Ultimately, it is a shallow framework of what *not* to do, without a more robust vision of what *can* be done, both for those with "slowly fatal conditions" and for those who have truly reached a terminal stage. It is a flawed, incomplete framework that we continue to promote. Instead of perpetuating this advance planning model, it may instead be time to reconfigure its foundations and focus.

CHALLENGES INHERENT
IN THE CURRENT CARE FRAMEWORK

Our current care system for patients with slowly progressing and ultimately fatal illness is really not a "system" at all. Rather, it usually consists of a haphazard, patchwork set of services linked together to manage the care of such patients as their needs evolve and they slowly progress toward the end of life. While managed care holds out the possibility for continuity of care and care planning across a spectrum of sites, and while recent initiatives have been developed to evaluate the efficacy and value of such continuity of care, the reality is that many patients still experience the choppy, event triggered, specialist driven late-life care evident in Rose's case. Decisions and care plans tends to be formulated and implemented to reflect circumstances of the moment, without considering longer term implications or anticipated changes in the symptoms and needs of the patient or the involved family. Not only is advance care planning for the end of life usually absent, but very frequently communication and planning across systems of care, or between the multitude of caregivers assisting the patient and family, is inadequate as well. Discontinuity of care and care planning continues to be the prevailing operational mode of our health care system.

In recent years evolving criteria and standards have emerged for pain and symptom management (Jacox, Car, Payne et al., 1994) and a literature has been developed describing gradual transitions in the goals of care as the patient enters a terminal stage (Doyle, 1997). Referral to a hospice program is considered to be an ideal approach once patients reach a late stage in their disease processes. Much of these guidelines and advice, however, have developed using cancer patients as the model, and thus there needs to be reconsideration and adaptation of such care guidelines for patients with other chronic and ultimately fatal diseases that have a more variable disease progression. Nonetheless, models of quality care for patients at the end of life now exist in the literature, in professional organizational pronouncements (Sachs, Ahronheim, Rhymes et al., 1995) and in select clinical consultation and service programs around the country (Portenoy, 1998; Walsh, 1990; Weissman & Griffee, 1994). How to get these guidelines and models integrated into a broader mainstream of clinical settings, however, is an ongoing challenge.

Nurturing and implementing new ways of conceptualizing care routines has historically been a Herculean challenge. Outdated standards of care die hard. Fiscal, regulatory, and organizational barriers frequently inhibit open-mindedness and innovation. Regarding end of life care, we are now at the point where significant differences in quality care practices and accessible services exist from one region of the country to another. For example, regional and geographic variations have now been documented for hospice utilization and the use of hospitalization at the very end of life (Wennberg & Cooper, 1998). Stark differences can even be found within the same geographic location. High quality pain management and palliative care services are developing within a short distance of facilities still utilizing outdated notions of pain management and dosing practices. Even in a single institution, the quality of a patient's end of life experience may depend enormously upon the service to which the patient is admitted and the training and inclination of the attending physician.

While not all patients desire hospice or have the option or interest in dying at home, it is likely that much of the differentiation in care patterns now evident at the end of life has more to do with inadequate training, misunderstanding, and outdated clinical concepts, rather than with actual patient choice. There are probably few patients, no matter what their care choices, who wish to die in pain, with inadequate symptom control, or in a humiliating, undignified state. It is therefore unjust, and indeed intolerable, that good pain management and symptom control can be the haphazard result of where one happens to live, who one's primary care physician is, or what care options a patient has chosen as life comes to a close. Whether or not one has the interest or ability to enter a quality hospice program, or instead chooses an aggressive but ultimately futile course of care, comfort and dignity should be available and integral to the care plan. The voices of advocacy on this issue need to be louder and stronger if we are to meet the coming demand portended by our changing demographics.

Despite strong efforts to improve public awareness and change professional attitudes, hospice programs continue to remain largely outside the mainstream clinical care for patients with late stage and end stage illness. There is no doubt that some of this continued estrangement results from the rigid regulatory and fiscal requirements built into the Medicare hospice benefit. The practices of some managed care organizations of further restricting hospice reimbursement is also a worrisome trend. At this time relatively few hospice programs are in a financial position to risk taking on patients with uncertain prognoses. Many hospices are confronted with very late, resource intensive referrals, which can likely only provide limited benefit to patients, and which expose these programs to the high up-front hospice admissions costs without the monetary balance derived from longer term reimbursement (Christakis and Escarce, 1996). It is unlikely that hospice referrals will substantially increase, or come much earlier, unless we can loosen the hospice admission criteria to consider severity of disease or symptoms, in addition to arbitrary prognostic time frames. But it is also unlikely that the impetus for such change will be strong enough unless demands for change echo in professional and public arenas far beyond the hospice community.

But even if progress is made and regulations are eased or loosened up, the question remains: if you build it, will they come? If hospice admission criteria regarding prognostication of terminality are eased, will more physicians recommend it? Will more patients seek it out?

There will likely still be the same kind of entrenched and blatant miseducation and misunderstanding about hospice that is prevalent in health care circles today. The comments of Rose's cardiologist concerning the target hospice patient population is a widely held misbelief, yet one often sustained by the fact that the majority of hospice patients continue to be patients with cancer diagnoses. Will hospice programs truly be ready and able to care for a large potential influx of slowing dying geriatric patients, whose own needs as well as their families' may be quite different from the more frequently encountered oncology patient? This is a question that hospice programs and clinicians will need to consider with candor and humility.

Moreover, just as there is a large percentage of the patient population who are constitutionally unable to consider planning in advance of incapacity and end of life, so there is also a certain percentage of the population who will never be able or willing to admit that the end of life is approaching, or that the chance for cure or restored functioning is non-existent. While they may accept and desire pain medication and relief of distressing symptoms, they may want little or nothing to do with what they perceive of as the hospice "philosophy." What is clear, then, is that there can be no one model of the "good death" against which all patients should be measured. Instead, we have to accept that patients of different persuasions, with different illnesses, of different cultures, and with differing values will define "a good death" on their own terms. Some of these patients would include and accept the hospice philosophy as a part of their definition, if only they knew about it. But many would not, and that point of view must be acceptable as well. What is not acceptable, however, is the lack of access and availability of quality palliative care for patients with late stage and end stage illness, no matter what their choices or setting of care. Whether or not Rose entered a hospice program, stayed at home, or was hospitalized, there was no excuse for the pain and suffering she endured as her life drew to a close.

SUGGESTIONS AND DIRECTIONS FOR CHANGE

The growth of our elderly population, and the chronicity, dementia, dependency and ultimately fatal illnesses that will follow, require a candid reconsideration of how we currently care for patients at the end of life, and what we need to do to improve that care. Specifically, we believe change and reconfiguration need to arise in at least two distinct areas: advance care planning and clinical training. Admittedly, any substantive reconsideration of these areas will require tremendous cooperation and collaboration across many disciplines and care settings. Furthermore, there are numerous administrative, regulatory, and fiscal hurdles that would need to be overcome in order to truly pave the way for change. The largest hurdle, however, comes not from outside the professional care communities but from within–from inadequate perceptions and attitudes about the experience of illness and the necessary decision framework for this patient population, and from limited cooperation and collaboration among all the disciplines that have a stake in this arena. Achieving change from outside will be hard, but pursuing change from within is inescapable.

Anticipatory Care Planning

Numerous studies and commentators have documented and described the many inadequacies of our current advance planning/advance directive framework (Teno, Stevens, Spernak & Lynn, 1998). The current autonomy-based framework has a conceptual focus of "prevention" and negation (preventing CPR, preventing feeding tubes, preventing ventilator use, etc.). What is equally essential when caring for patients with slowly fatal conditions is a companion conceptual framework that is pro-active and anticipatory–not of what should be avoided, but rather of what *can* be anticipated, planned for and embraced, in a positive, proactive way. The current advance directive framework gives clinicians a rather shallow set of obligations–that is, ensure that certain interventions *don't* happen to the patient. But shouldn't there also be more positive obligations that clinicians intrinsically accept when such patients are under their care?

It may be important for a newly diagnosed cardiac patient to select a health care proxy, and to consider whether or not she would want to be resuscitated at a late stage in the illness. But for patients with heart conditions or other slowly fatal conditions, it is equally if not more important to be able to anticipate what will be the symptoms and signposts along the way–what might the continuum of decline look like, prior to the very end of life, and what are the care options in response? For example, it seemed as though no one discussed with Rose what her life might be like in the months before that final hospitalization. Was she aware of the many other important considerations beyond health care proxies and DNR orders? Did she know that a palliative approach, with much earlier hospice referral, was an option? In essence, what is needed for patients like Rose is not simply end of life care planning, but rather a *continuum* of considerations and decision making in anticipation of an eventually fatal outcome. Planning for the end of life should not be truncated from the living that leads to that end.

This type of planning necessarily involves collaboration and connection across the settings in which patients receive care as their health deteriorates. It places positive obligations on clinicians to work with patients and families so they can anticipate what may be coming and what the available options are in response. In this anticipatory planning framework broad parameters of care options and patient values are sketched out and articulated in advance, while ongoing and regular dialogue shapes the specific decisions and options as particular symptoms set in. We know that the experience of illness may change attitudes and tolerance, and priorities may be reconfigured as disease progresses and options become more clear. This is a framework that anticipates needs and options yet also recognizes that as illness progresses, the dynamics of change may critically influence care choices and delivery.

Such anticipatory planning must be more than just a catalogue of possible physical symptoms. It is important for patients and their intimate caregivers to understand what physical changes may appear and how needs and caregiving may change in response. There are, however, many other considerations that are critical to this anticipatory planning. A more robust array of considerations might include the following: anticipated changes in functional capacity and the patient's ability to be independent; anticipated pain or other distressing symptoms that may require palliative care as a companion to other sorts of interventions (and that may naturally lead to a hospice referral); foreseeable mental status changes, including dementia, delirium, or other psychological responses caused by the illness; potential changes in familial/caregiving responsibilities and time commitments; possible changes in the appropriate setting of care, or the need for formally paid caregivers; medication changes and their anticipated side-effects; religious, spiritual or other existential considerations that may take on more meaning or urgency as a patient progresses more deeply into illness; anticipatory grieving or other emotional responses of the patient or family as they begin to face an impending loss; and foreseeable legal or financial considerations that may arise from diminished capacity, or increased functional dependence.

Within this rich anticipatory framework, consideration of hospice should naturally arise in the course of continuing dialogue, rather than suddenly emerge as a sharply divergent alternative when "there is nothing more to be done." With a planning framework that anticipates along a continuum of disease progression, hospice referral may occur much earlier than currently happens. The holistic approach of hospice care fits squarely within the broader array of considerations critical to this anticipatory framework. Discussion of hospice would be a natural, indeed essential, component to the ongoing anticipation of needs and options. Ideally, through this framework, pain and symptom management, functional concerns, and attention to familial and emotional needs will have been essential considerations at points all along the disease projectory. Hospice as a care option, therefore, will not appear as a foreign or feared alternative: rather, it will be a comfortable continuation of the comprehensive view of patient care and caring already in place. Not all patients and families will embrace hospice as an acceptable care option as chronic illness progresses. But with this framework, all will appreciate why the option exists and how it might be of benefit.

This will not be an easy advance care framework to capture on a form or to reconfigure into a set of boxes to be checked off. It certainly cannot be adequately addressed in a five minute conversation or even in a single clinical visit. It anticipates a continuum of conversation with a fluid and flexible framework. It is a more robust framework of anticipated needs and care'options than our current configurations of advance care planning, as it more accurately considers the *person* who is the patient. In a more comprehensive way it captures the day to day experiences that patients and families endure as they move inevitably, though perhaps not imminently, toward the end of life. This framework does not negate the need for consideration of such dramatic options as CPR (cardiopulminary resuscitation), feeding tubes or ventilatory support. Acute crisis or sudden incapacity can never be fully anticipated. But it moves well beyond the "negative" autonomy paradigm as our sole, guiding value. Rather, for clinicians it creates positive obligations as well: through ongoing dialogue, they must bring the virtues of caring and continuous commitment to this advance planning process, no matter what the course of disease or choice of the patient.

New Concepts of Clinical Training

In order for this more robust, anticipatory planning framework to resonate among clinicians and become integrated into routine clinical care patterns, physicians and others who care for patients like Rose must have the knowledge to anticipate into the future and the competency to address what may arise. While this does not mean that every primary care physician must be a specialist in geriatric medicine, or that every cardiologist must be a palliative care expert, what it does underscore is a minimum level of basic competency that all who care for elderly patients with slowly fatal conditions must possess. At a minimum they must possess the awareness to anticipate potential symptoms, the communication skills to conduct candid discussions of care options, and the assessment skills to know when to refer to specialists. While not all physicians can be expected to be pain specialists, for example, it is unconscionable that in this day and age there are still physicians who do not anticipate or assess for pain, and who do not consult with pain specialists when appropriate.

What this suggests is the need for "blended competencies" among those who care for this patient population. That is, medical school curricula and residency training programs must acknowledge the skills necessary to care for such patients and create training opportunities in response. For example, programs combining residency training in oncology and geriatrics have been suggested, recognizing the particular symptoms and needs specific to the older cancer population (Bennett, Sahasrabudhe & Hall, 1997). As well, the ongoing shortage of physicians trained through accredited geriatric fellowship programs has underscored the need to teach basic aspects of geriatric medicine to internal and primary care physicians, relying on specially trained geriatricians only in cases demanding more advanced expertise (Rimer, 1998). We have arrived at a point in time where it is simply unacceptable that basic training in geriatrics is an elective for most physicians, or that the fundamentals of palliative care are considered optional for virtually all physicians in training. The likelihood is that few physicians in practice today will escape the reality of caring for such patients as their patient populations age, and few patients and families will escape the reality of this progressive disease course. Why, then, aren't the basic fundamentals of caring for these patients considered integral to most training programs?

Interestingly, both the field of geriatrics and the emerging field of palliative care promote similar goals and face similar obstacles: Both fields view the patient and her circumstances within a broader perspective than simply a set of medical conditions or physical symptoms. Both utilize an interdisciplinary approach to patient care that includes consideration of the social and emotional circumstances of the patient, and the family constellation that supports or complicates care goals. Both understand the essential role of planning and anticipation, and the need for strong communication skills to support such efforts. However, both fields face the challenge of ensuring that primary care physicians and disease specialists have the basic knowledge and clinical skills necessary to adequately care for these patients, yet also ensure that they have in their possession the awareness and assessment skills necessary to know when consultation or transfer to a specialist is appropriate. While a few savvy patients and their families may take the initiative to seek out geriatricians or palliative care specialists on their own, the reality is that most access to these specialties will come through primary care or disease specialist referrals. This is especially true as managed care systems tighten access to specialists through the use of primary care physicians. Teaching such physicians basic aspects of geriatric and palliative care is thus essential to ensuring quality primary care for these patients, and to opening up access to these specialties when appropriate.

Collaborative advocacy among palliative care specialists and geriatric professionals may be an especially useful approach, then, in efforts to reconfigure clinical training programs and create access to quality care for patients with slowly fatal conditions. Such collaborative advocacy should be fully interdisciplinary, including the array of professionals whose valuable skills and perspectives combine to encompass quality geriatric and palliative patient care. Hospice in particular has a critical role in such advocacy efforts: not only must hospice clinicians work to increase awareness and understanding of hospice within the larger, mainstream medical community, but they must also work more closely with colleagues from the geriatric community to help ensure better understanding and better continuity of care for elderly patients with eventually fatal diseases. In turn, professionals from the geriatric community must work to ensure that hospice and palliative care specialists have a clear understanding of what particular needs and concerns may accompany the elderly patient with slowly fatal disease, in contrast to the more commonly encountered oncology patient. Each discipline has an extraordinary opportunity to expand the horizon of the other, and, in collaboration, to help lead efforts to improve access to quality care for all patients at the end of life and their families, no matter what their illness or setting of care.

It would, of course, be naive to assume that more creative training programs will solve our problems concerning access to quality care for patients with slowly fatal conditions. A multifaceted, relentless approach will be necessary. For example, it is clear the clinicians' attitudes and practice patterns are highly influenced by clinical mentoring and the culture of their clinical setting. Thus, collaborative advocacy must go beyond the classroom and into the trenches: modeling of quality patient assessment and support for quality end of life care must be visible to all who deal with this patient population. Examples of quality conversations and robust anticipatory planning must be modeled by those with the expertise for all those who need to acquire it. While there is an ongoing need to help patients and their families become savvy medical consumers, especially regarding end of life care, there is an equal urgency that clinicians themselves create the climate of conversation necessary to truly engage in a robust dialogue along the continuum of disease and decline.

Beyond the clinical community this collaborative advocacy needs to extend into the policy arena and the legislative halls. While recognizing the need to upgrade clinical skills and alter clinical attitudes, we must also have systems of care delivery and financing that acknowledge and provide access to quality palliative care no matter what kind of care patients with slowly fatal diseases desire, and no matter what their setting of care. Reimbursement schema and quality of care monitoring must be reconfigured to adjust to what is now recognized as the standard of care that ought to be available to all patients in such circumstances. Access to quality pain management and symptom alleviation ought to be available to all patients with slowly fatal conditions, whether they reside in the community, find themselves in a hospital or eventually seek the services of a long term care facility. For some of these patients, earlier referral to hospice will provide that necessary access to care. For others, changes in the current hospice admission criteria to account for severity of disease rather than arbitrary prognostic models will be necessary. And for others, entrance into a hospice program will be undesirable or unattainable–but that should be no excuse for less than quality attention to the needs and concerns that patients experience as they transition to the end stage of their lives. It is simply no longer tolerable that our systems of financing care and structuring care delivery for these elderly patients serve as barriers, rather than facilitators, of quality care at the end of life.

CONCLUSION

While the care provided to Rose reminds us all of how far we have to go, we should not lose sight of how far we have truly come. We no longer live in a society that tries to deny death. Meaningful dialogue about care of the dying and exploration of creative opportunities to improve the end of life are evident in both professional and lay communities, even as we simultaneously strategize about how to more "successfully age." While few of us unambiguously embrace the end of life, most of us have now gained the experiential wisdom that inevitably accompanies the "bad" death of a loved one or a favorite patient, and that shocks us into recognition that for our patients, our loved ones, and for ourselves, we would want something "better." The challenge is how to mobilize that self-awareness of what constitutes "dying well" into concrete advocacy to promote change, and how to build and sustain the infrastructure to support it.

A sense of urgency, indeed emergency, is not out of place in this discussion. The aging population is exploding, and soon enough "they" will be "we." For better or worse, almost all of us will join the ranks of this growing geriatric population. We may be successful at aging, but none of us will successfully avoid dying. Therefore, the one strong goal we should all work toward, no matter what our care perspective or setting, is that we collaboratively and successfully build a future where the pain and suffering experienced by Rose is no longer even a possibility. After all, though our journeys may be different, the end of life awaits us all.

REFERENCES

Bennett, J.M., Sahasrabudhe, D.M. & Hall, W.J. (1997). Medical oncology and geriatric medicine: Is it time for fellowship integration? *Cancer*, 80(7), 1351-1353.

Cassel, C.K. & Siegel, L.C. (1998). *Medicare for the 21st century: The goals of health coverage for our aging society.* Report commissioned by the National Academy of Social Insurance in support of its Restructuring Medicare for the Long Term Project.

Christakis, N.A. & Escarce, J.J. (1996). Survival of Medicare patients After Enrollment in Hospice Programs. *New England Journal of Medicine* 335(3): 172-178.

Cicirelli, V.G. (1997). Elders' end-of-life decisions: Implications for hospice care. *The Hospice Journal*, 12(1), 57-72.

Cleary, J.F. & Carbone, P.P. (1997). Palliative medicine in the elderly. *Cancer*, 80(7), 1335-1347.

Doyle, D. (1997). "The provision of palliative care," in Doyle, D., Hanks, G.W.C. & MacDonald, N. Oxford *Textbook of Palliative Medicine* (2nd edition). Oxford: Oxford University Press.

Dubler, N.N. (1995). The doctor-proxy relationship: The neglected connection. *Kennedy Institute of Ethics Journal*, 5, 280-306.

Fischer, G.S., Tulsky, J.A., Rose, M.R. et al. (1998). Patient knowledge and physician predictions of treatment preferences after discussion of advance directives. *Journal of General Internal Medicine*, 13(7), 447-454.

Hare, J., Pratt, C. & Nelson, C. (1992). Agreement between patients and their self-selected surrogates on difficult medical decisions. *Archives of Internal Medicine*, 152 (5), 1049-1054.

Institute of Medicine, Committee on Care at the End of Life (1997). *Approaching Death: Improving Care at the End of Life.* Washington, D.C: National Academy Press.

Jacox, A., Car, D.B., Payne, R. et al. (1994). *Management of Cancer Pain.* Clinical Practice Guideline No. 9. AHCPR Publication No. 94-0592. Rockville, MD: Agency for Health Care Policy and Research, U.S. Dept. of Health and Human Services, Public Health Service.

Levine, C. & Zuckerman, C. (1999). The trouble with families: Toward and ethic of accommodation. *Annals of Internal Medicine, 130: 148-152.*

Lynn, J. (1997). An 88-year old woman facing the end of life. *Journal of the American Medical Association*, 277 (20), 1633-1640.

Lynn, J. & Teno, J. (1993). After the Patient Self-Determination Act: The need for empirical research on formal advance directives. *The Hastings Center Report*, 23(1), 20-24.

The Omnibus Budget Reconciliation Act of 1990, Pub.L. 101-508, Section 4206, 4751 (OBRA), 42 U.S.C. Section 1395cc(f)(1) & 42 U.S.C. Section 1396a(a) (Supp. 1991).

Portenoy, R.K. (Nov., 1998), "Expanding the scope of care: Moving from pain management to palliative care," presentation at the 17th Annual Scientific Meeting of the American Pain Society, San Diego, CA.

Rimer, Sara (Sept. 24, 1998). Medicine's new frontier: Treating the elderly. *The New York Times*, A1, Col. 4.

Sachs, G.A., Ahronheim, J.C., Rhymes, J.A. et al. (1995). Good care of dying patients: The alternative to physician-assisted suicide and euthanasia. *Journal of the American Geriatrics Society*, 43, 553-562.

Sengstaken, E.A. & King, S.A. (1993) The problems of pain and its detection among geriatric nursing home residents. *Journal of the American Geriatrics Society*, 41, 541-544.

Suhl, J., Simons, P., Reedy, T. & Garrick, T. (1994). Myth of Substituted Judgment. *Archives of Internal Medicine,* 154, 90-96.

Teno, J., Licks, S., Lynn, J. et al. (1997). Do advance directives provide instructions that direct care? *Journal of the American Geriatrics Society,* 45(4), 508-512.

Teno, J., Stevens, M., Spernak, S. & Lynn, J. (1998). Role of written advance directives in decision making: insights from qualitative and quantitative data. *Journal of General Internal Medicine,* 13(7), 439-446.

Walsh, T.D. (1990). Continuing Care in a Medical Center: The Cleveland Clinic Foundation Palliative Care Service. *Journal of Pain and Symptom Management,* 5(5), 273-278.

Weissman, D.E. & Griffee, J. (1994). The Palliative Care Consultation Service of the Medical College of Wisconsin. *Journal of Pain and Symptom Management,* 9(7), 474-479.

Wennberg, J.E. & Cooper, M.M. (1998). *The Dartmouth Atlas of Health Care.* Chicago: American Hospital Publishing, pp. 81-106.

CURRENT EFFORTS

End-of-Life Care:
Challenges and Opportunities
for Health Care Professionals

Deborah Witt Sherman

SUMMARY. The failings of the American Health Care System in meeting the comprehensive needs of the seriously and terminally ill have led to both professional and public efforts to improve end-of-life care. Following a discussion of the shortcomings of end-of-life in America, this article describes the goals and philosophy of palliative care, while highlighting current innovative programs in end-of-life needs and insure quality of life for patients and families experiencing incurable, progressive illness. Health care professionals are called to respond to the challenges and opportunities of end-of-life care as individual health care providers, as members of professions, and as members of interdisciplinary teams committed to improving the care of the dying in America. *[Article copies available for a fee from The Haworth Document Delivery Service: 1-800-342-9678. E-mail address: getinfo@haworthpressinc. com <Website: http://www.haworthpressinc.com>]*

KEYWORDS. End-of-life, palliative care, health care professionals

---

[Haworth co-indexing entry note]: "End-of-Life Care: Challenges and Opportunities for Health Care Professionals." Sherman, Deborah Witt. Co-published simultaneously in *The Hospice Journal* (The Haworth Press, Inc.) Vol. 14, No. 3/4, 1999, pp. 109-121; and: *The Hospice Heritage: Celebrating Our Future* (ed: Inge B. Corless and Zelda Foster) The Haworth Press, Inc., 1999, pp. 109-121. Single or multiple copies of this article are available for a fee from The Haworth Document Delivery Service [1-800-342-9678, 9:00 a.m. - 5:00 p.m. (EST). E-mail address: getinfo@haworthpressinc.com].

End-of-life care provides challenges and opportunities for all health care professionals. Acknowledging their unique contributions, health care professionals must learn to work effectively as members of an interdisciplinary team whose unified purpose is to secure the best possible quality of life of patients and families facing incurable, progressive, and terminal illness. Documentation of the shortcomings of end-of-life care in America was a rude awakening as to the failings of the American health care system in meeting the comprehensive needs of the terminally ill (Cunningham, 1997). Uncomfortable with a failing report card, the public and health care institutions have initiated a concerted effort to improve the care of the dying in America.

The Hospice movement serves as the template for effective and compassionate end-of-life care. Hospice philosophy and principles provide the foundation for the emerging specialty of palliative care, which has taken a broader perspective in addressing the comprehensive needs of patients along all points of the illness trajectory. The goals and precepts of palliative care acknowledge the need for an interdisciplinary perspective, yet each health care discipline must assume responsibility in assuring that its profession is doing everything possible to alleviate suffering at the end-of-life and provide a respectful death. The recent position statement by nursing on the inclusion of pain assessment as the fifth vital sign is one example of nursing's active role in end-of-life care (A Peaceful Death Symposium, University of North Carolina at Chapel Hill, December 3rd, 1998). This article provides a context to understand the challenges and opportunities for all health care professionals regarding end-of-life care in America and hopefully will stimulate a discussion among professionals of "What can be done by tomorrow?" to improve the care of the dying.

SHORTCOMINGS OF END-OF-LIFE CARE IN AMERICA

The report card on end-of-life care in America indicated the failing marks of medical institutions. Such marks were based on the results of the SUPPORT study (1995), which was funded by the Robert Wood Johnson Foundation, and involved five leading medical institutions in the United States and nearly 10,000 critically ill patients. The results indicated the frequency of aggressive treatment at the end-of-life, and physicians' lack of knowledge regarding patients' end-of-life wishes. In addition, less than half the Do Not Resuscitate (DNR) orders were written within two days of death, over one-third of the patients spent their last days in the Intensive Care Units (ICU), half of the patients died in moderate to severe pain, and there was a consistent lack of communication between patients and their physicians. In the second phase of the study, brief interventions by specially trained nurses to inform physicians about the patient's preferences for treatment and reminders about the patients' need for pain management resulted in no significant difference in physicians' behaviors and end-of-life outcomes.

The results of the SUPPORT study underscored the findings of Chernyl, Coyle, and Foley (1993) and highlighted the need for more effective pain and symptom management to alleviate all dimensions of suffering at the end of life. Their taxonomy of suffering identified the common shortcomings of end-of-life care in America, including inadequate control of pain and other symptoms; undiagnosed depression; anxiety and existential distress; untreated psychological distress and fatigue in family members; and lack of effective communication particularly where cultural differences exist. Having invested 28 million dollars in the SUPPORT study, the Robert Wood Johnson Foundation (RWJ) extended its commitment to end-of-life care by launching several major initiatives which recognize the "overriding need to change the kind of care dying Americans receive" (Robert Wood Johnson Foundation Last Acts, 1996).

IDENTIFYING THE GOALS
AND PRECEPTS OF PALLIATIVE CARE

The remedial work of the Robert Wood Johnson Foundation began with the Last Acts Campaign to engage both professionals and the public in efforts to improve end-of-life care. As the first step in achieving end-of-life reform, the Last Acts Task Force (1998) developed a set of core precepts that identify the goals of palliative care and provide a foundation for developing new strategies for palliative care. Fundamental to these precepts is the definition of palliative care. Palliative care has been defined as a philosophy of care that involves a combination of active and compassionate therapies intended to support and comfort individuals and families who are living with life threatening illness. The goal of palliative care is to achieve the best quality of life by meeting the physical, psychological, social, spiritual and existential expectations and needs of patients while remaining sensitive to personal, cultural, and religious beliefs, values, and practices (Last Acts Task Force, 1998).

The precepts of palliative care therefore involve: (1) a respect for patient goals, preferences and choices; (2) comprehensive caring which addresses the holistic needs of patients and alleviates isolation through a commitment to non-abandonment and ongoing communication; (3) acknowledging and addressing caregiver concerns and the need for supportive services; (4) utilizing the strengths of interdisciplinary resources; and (5) the development of institutional infrastructures that support best practices and models of palliative care (Last Acts Task Force, 1998).

The strategies for change proposed by the Last Acts Campaign include (1) improving communication and decision making, specifically by creating opportunities and methods for talking about death and dying, recognition of death as a natural process, and the value of advanced directives, as well as improving communication skills of health professionals; (2) changing health care and health care institutions by strengthening professional education related to end-of-life care; making palliative care an integral part of patient care; developing benchmarks to evaluate palliative care; broadening insurance coverage of palliative care and counseling; incorporating successes of the Hospice movement into other health care settings; and identifying other models for compassionate and effective end-of-life care; as well as (3) changing American culture and attitudes towards death and dying while recognizing the diverse needs of patients and families from various cultures and religious traditions; making information on death and dying available to the public; and facilitating open discussions with special educational efforts on families (Robert Wood Johnson Foundation Last Acts, 1996).

These objectives can only be accomplished through a concerted effort by all health care disciplines and by the public's awareness of the importance of such efforts, their receptivity to changing the societal perspectives of death, and the recognition of death as a natural part of the life process. Involvement of the public has created numerous initiatives related to end-of-life care, giving momentum to a new movement to improve the care of dying Americans.

END-OF-LIFE MOVEMENT–
THE CALL FOR INNOVATIVE PROGRAMS
IN END-OF-LIFE CARE

"Until recently, medicine has been obsessed with new technology for saving lives. The goal of prolonging life, or equivalently, fighting against death, defined the path of medicine . . . Today, medicine seems to be moving on a new path toward a more balanced view of its role in death and dying . . . in the direction of helping patients die well" (Connelly, 1998, p. 332). The new path suggested by Connelly is being selected in an attempt to clarify seriously ill patients' preferences, improve decision making at the end-of-life, help health care professionals use advanced medical technology more judiciously, particularly when it no longer serves the patient's best interests, and relieve patients' pain and discomfort (Cunningham, 1997).

The repercussions of the SUPPORT study has led to a new movement to target the shortcomings in end-of-life care. The major components of the movement include:

- The $15-million Project on Death in America which has funded end-of-life programs and fellowships and brought together many other foundations to coordinate efforts in end-of-life care;
- The Center to Improve the Care of the Dying, located in Washington D.C., which has launched initiatives including the compilation of a "Sourcebook on Dying" which provides scientific knowledge on end-of-life care; preparation of a Toolkit to measure end-of-life outcomes; as well as the development of a new health care policy called Medicaring in which a select population of Medicare patients would shift their Medicare resources from potentially futile medical interventions toward comprehensive, supportive, community-based services;
- The Institute of Medicine's End-of-Life Committee which has issued a two volume report, published as a text entitled "Approaching Death: Improving Care at the End-of-Life," concluding that end-of-life care is an important responsibility of health care providers and which emphasized the need to reform prescription laws to insure effective pain management for dying patients, as well as identifying other important practice, research, and educational initiatives related to end-of-life care;

- The American Medical Association which has launched a two-year project called Education for Physicians in End-of-Life Care (EPEC), funded by RWJ, to train physicians in end-of-life care; and
- The Missoula Demonstration Project in Montana began a 15-year initiative to introduce the dialogue about death and dying in the community, identify what dying well really means, and document the findings (Cunningham, 1997).

THE CONTRIBUTIONS
OF THE HOSPICE MOVEMENT
TO PALLIATIVE CARE AND ITS DISTINCTIONS

"The Hospice movement has contributed to clearing a new path in medicine" (Connelly, 1998, p. 333)–a path which assists individuals in dying well. Clearly, Hospice has advocated for a holistic philosophy of care that responds to the physical, psychological, social, and spiritual needs of dying patients and their families and the appropriate use of medications in the alleviation of pain and suffering.

Palliative care has its origins in Hospice care, which originated in London in 1967 through the work of Dame Cicely Saunders. As a nurse, social worker, and physician, she understood the complex interdisciplinary needs of dying patients. The principles of Hospice care set forth by Saunders included the patient's acceptance of death; care managed by an interdisciplinary team; the control of common symptoms of disease, especially pain; recognition of patient and family as a single unit; and implementation of home care for the dying and bereavement care for the family after the patient's death (Sheehan & Forman, 1996).

Today, Hospice care may be viewed as a specific model for delivering palliative care or as a subset of palliative care (Byock, 1998). While both Hospice and palliative care provide a holistic focus and an interdisciplinary approach, differences do exist. For example, the eligibility for Hospice care requires a prognosis of 6 months or less to live while palliative Care extends across the disease trajectory; Hospice Care expects the acknowledgment of death by patient and family while palliative care does not have the absolute connotation of dying; and Hospice care involves no curative treatments while palliative care may involve curative and supportive treatment, as well as prevention strategies (Sheehan & Forman, 1996).

AGGRESSIVE COMFORT TREATMENTS: ADDRESSING END-OF-LIFE NEEDS AND INSURING QUALITY OF LIFE

A challenge of end-of-life care is to educate health care professionals in recognizing the need for aggressive comfort care in alleviating suffering and to acquire the related skills and competencies in providing palliative care. The end-of-life needs of patients reflect physical concerns (pain and symptoms), psychological distress (depression and existential anxiety), limitations in functioning (physical, emotional, and social), spiritual distress, as well as issues related to social support, promoting the health care provider-patient relationship, and planning for preferences in end-of-life care (Fields & Cassel, 1997). In addressing these needs, palliative care focuses on the individual's right to be informed; respect for the patient and family's needs regarding the sharing of information, timely access to information and services in a language that can be understood; the availability of palliative care services 24 hours a day, seven days a week; the assurance of confidentiality; and the commitment that continuity of care will be offered by an interdisciplinary team of caregivers working collaboratively with the individual and family (Ferris et al., 1995).

An important understanding is that palliative care does not imply that "there is nothing more that can be done" but rather that a team of experts will take a positive approach, focusing on what can and will be done for dying patients and their families. Murphy and Price (1995) call this care "ACT," a mnemonic for "Aggressive Comfort Treatment." This approach encompasses the precepts of hospice care, as the patient and family understand the continued commitment of health care professionals to holistic care and the attempt to alleviate all dimensions of suffering–physical, emotional, social, and spiritual. The opportunity for patients and families to actively participate in end-of-life choices and decision making in accordance with their values, beliefs, and preferences promotes a sense of hopefulness, and diminishes a sense of helplessness. The opportunity for treatment options in positive terms and comfort-oriented care for dying patients emphasizes that everything possible will be done to promote quality of life until death.

The effectiveness of the initiatives to promote comprehensive and compassionate end-of-life care must be determined by measurements of the dimensions of quality of life for patients and their family caregivers. Quality of life includes physical well-being, emotional well-being, social well-being, health and functioning, spirituality, and treatment satisfaction (Aaronson, 1990; Cella & Tulsky, 1990; Ferrans & Powers, 1995). In addition, King et al. (1997) suggest that access to the primary care provider, socioeconomic status, the delivery of health services, and social support be measured as additional dimensions of quality of life in the context of serious illness. Financial burden on the family, and bereavement and grief resolution are also added dimensions of quality of life of the family (Stewart, Teno, Patrick, & Lynn, 1998). Critically evaluating quality of life outcomes for patients and families provides an opportunity for health professionals to distinguish excellent from merely adequate palliative care and to take corrective actions when necessary within the context of an interdisciplinary team.

INTERDISCIPLINARY APPROACH TO HOSPICE AND PALLIATIVE CARE

The ability of Hospice care and palliative care to meet the comprehensive physical, psychological, social, and spiritual needs of patients and families is dependent on the interdisciplinary work of physicians, nurses, social workers, clergy, dieticians, pharmacists, and physical, occupational, and music therapists. The formation of a team implies a common purpose and identity whose goals are to maximize therapies that minimize distress and improve the quality of life for patients and families (Sheehan & Forman, 1997). The interdisciplinary team for end-of-life care assists patients and families in defining the goals of care and effectively mobilizes each other's skills to meet patient's needs across a variety of health care settings, including inpatient palliative units or palliative care consultation teams, inpatient Hospice programs, community-based Hospice programs, skilled nursing facilities' Hospice programs, and home-based Hospice care.

The interdisciplinary approach is different from a multidisciplinary approach where the individual identities of the team members supersede that of a team identity and there is less opportunity for formal group communication regarding patient and family preferences, expectations, and response to care (Sheehan & Forman, 1997). The need for an interdisciplinary approach to care occurs when there is deterio-ration of the patient's health evident by multiple symptoms, decreas-ing functional status, increasing emotional or spiritual distress, ad-vancing disease which is not responding to therapies, as well as increasing burden or stress placed on the family. The palliative care model therefore stresses the humanistic qualities of the patient, the family, and care providers and alleviates suffering within the context of these intrapersonal and interpersonal relationships.

NURSING'S INITIATIVES REGARDING END-OF-LIFE CARE

Throughout its history, nursing has ministered to the needs of the dying, relieving not only the pain and symptoms associated with in-curable and progressive diseases, but attending to emotional and spiri-tual needs of patients and families at the end-of-life. In 1995, the American Nurses Association (ANA) reaffirmed a position statement on the promotion of comfort and relief of pain in dying patients. In summary, the ANA stated that it is the nurse's obligation to promote comfort and insure aggressive efforts to relieve the pain and symptoms of dying patients. Furthermore, it was stated that increasing the titra-tion of medication to achieve adequate symptom control, even at the expense of life, thus hastening death secondarily, is ethically justified (American Nurses Association, 1995). While this statement strongly supports nursing's role in end-of-life care, education has been needed to dispel the myths regarding opioid addiction in the context of end-of-life care.

The results of the SUPPORT study have provided evidence that all health professionals need to take active roles in improving the care of the dying. The need to improve nursing education regarding end-of-life care has been acknowledged. Under the auspices of the American Association of Colleges of Nurses and supported by RWJ (November, 1997), a roundtable of nursing experts was convened in Washington, DC to discuss undergraduate nursing care competencies regarding end-of-life. A document entitled "Peaceful Death: Recommended Competencies and Curricular Guidelines for End-of-Life Nursing Care," now available on the Internet, was developed to outline bacca-laureate competencies for end-of-life care and content areas where competencies can be taught (Internet, <http:\\www.aacn.nche.edu\SpecProj\index.html>). This document has been disseminated to all baccalaureate nursing programs in the country.

The initiative to educate graduate nurses in palliative care has been led by New York University (NYU) which has implemented the first Advanced Practice Nurse Practitioner Master's Program in Palliative Care in the United States and by Ursuline College in Ohio which has implemented an Advanced Practice Clinical Nurse Specialist Program in Palliative Care. NYU's Program has been funded by the United States Department of Health and Human Services, and as program director, Dr. Deborah Witt Sherman has been funded by the Soros Foundation as a Project on Death in America Faculty Scholar to carry out this initiative.

NYU's Palliative Care Practitioner Program builds on the core curriculum of the Master's program, focusing on theory, research, critical thinking, human development, community and leadership. In addition to advanced courses in pathophysiology, pharmacotherapeutics, and advanced health assessment, student's curriculum include a role development course and five specialized courses in palliative care that include content on loss, grief, death and bereavement, advanced care planning, legal and ethical issues at the end-of-life, spirituality, health provider-patient communication, pain and symptom management, skills in leading interdisciplinary teams, and support groups, as well as nursing's role in the development of health care policies and standards of practice for palliative care. The program also includes 710 precepted clinical hours.

Recently, the responsibility of nursing in improving end-of-life care has been recognized by the leaders of the American Nurses Association, the American Association of Colleges of Nurses, the National League of Nursing, the American Academy of Nurses, and the International Council of Nurses at a symposium sponsored by the Robert Wood Johnson Foundation and entitled "A Peaceful Death" at the University of North Carolina, Chapel Hill (December 3rd, 1998). Within the context of an interdisciplinary forum, nurse leaders and others stressed the importance of an interdisciplinary approach to palliative care. However, given the history of nursing, its focus on holistic care, and proximity to patients and families, a consensus was reached and a position statement was formulated regarding nurses' responsibility for end-of-life care. The statement reads as follows:

> An important part of nursing responsibility is to improve end-of-life care for all. To that end, nurse leaders will launch an initiative

to incorporate pain assessment as the fifth (5th) vital sign, along with temperature, pulse, respiration, and blood pressure and nurses will take appropriate action. Further, nursing and nurses will assume responsibility for end-of-life care and assemble the appropriate interdisciplinary team. (A Peaceful Death Symposium University of North Carolina, December 3rd, 1998)

The significance of this statement is that nursing assumes an active role in creating an interdisciplinary approach to improve end-of-life care. The coordinated efforts of all members of the interdisciplinary team will improve the patient's quality of life until its end and promote a respectful death.

EMERGING POSSIBILITIES IN END-OF-LIFE CARE– INTERDISCIPLINARY EDUCATIONAL INITIATIVES

The question for new palliative care programs will be whether they reflect best practices in Hospice care contingent on a set of values of quality of care and an orientation to patients and families (Byock, 1998). Best practices in Hospice/palliative care lies within the context of an interdisciplinary approach to care as no one health care profession alone is able to meet the broad range of needs of people at the end-of-life. Furthermore, the economic reality is that efficient health care can only be achieved by an interdisciplinary effort. At this point in time, the degree of palliative care education that exists is discipline specific and often limited. There is little in the education of health professionals that prepares them to work collaboratively in providing palliative care. The result is that clinical time is often consumed by professionals learning to work together through trial and error.

The Last Acts Task Force (1998) therefore recommends the strengthening of education of health care professionals related to death, dying, and end-of-life care, and the Institute of Medicine (IOM) recommends the initiation of changes in undergraduate, graduate, and continuing education that improve the knowledge, attitudes, and skills in end-of-life care. Furthermore, the IOM suggests that palliative care become a defined area of expertise, education, and research (Fields & Cassel, 1997). The Robert Wood Johnson Foundation supports proposals for interdisciplinary educational initiatives to insure collaborative efforts of all health disciplines involved in palliative care so that comprehensive, patient-centered care will be available to all individuals facing the end-of-life. The quality of care at the end-of-life clearly depends on the education of health care professionals who have clinical knowledge, technical skills, competency in interpersonal skills and a respect for individuals' values, beliefs and preferences.

CONCLUSION

The challenges and opportunities in end-of-life care are before us as health care professionals. We must ask ourselves, "What can be done by tomorrow to make a difference in the lives of individuals and families facing death?" Each of us may begin with a questioning of our own personal perspectives and values related to death and dying and end-of-life care, followed by a question of what each profession can do to insure quality care at the end-of-life, and lastly, what we can do as an interdisciplinary team of health professionals to insure that the failures evident by the SUPPORT study will be corrected.

REFERENCES

Aaronson, N. (1990). Quality of life research in cancer clinical trials: A need for common rules and language. *Oncology*, 4, 59-66.

American Association of Colleges of Nursing. (November, 1997). *Peaceful death.* Internet: <http://www.aacn.nche.edu/Index/SpecProj>.

American Nurses Association (1995). *Position statement on promotion of comfort and relief of pain in dying patients.* Washington, D.C.: American Nurses Publishing.

Byock, I. (1998). Hospice and palliative care: A parting of ways or a path to the future? *Journal of Palliative Medicine*, 1(2), 165-176.

Cella, D. F., & Tulsky, D. S. (1990). Measuring quality of life today: Methodological aspects. *Oncology*, 4, 29-38.

Chernyl, N. I., Coyle, N., & Foley, K. (1994). Suffering in the advanced cancer patient: A definition and taxonomy. *Journal of Palliative Care*, 10(2), 54-57.

Connelly, R. J. (1998). The medicalization of dying: A positive turn on a new path. Omega, 36(4), 331-341.

Cunningham, R. (1997). End-of-life movement targets care shortcomings. *Medicine & Health Perspectives*, (November, 3), 1-4.

Ferrans, C., & Power, M. (1995). Quality of Life Index: Development and psychometric properties. *Advances in Nursing Sciences*, 8, 15-24.

Ferris, F., Flannery, J., McNeal, H., Morissette, M., Camerons, R., & Bally, G. (1995). *Palliative care: A comprehensive guide for the care of persons with HIV disease.* Ontario, Canada: Mount Sinai Hospital/Casey House Hospice, 1995.

Fields, M., & Cassel, C. (1997). *Approaching death: Improving care at the end-of-life.* Washington, D.C.: National Academy Press.

King, C., Haberman, M., Berry, D., Bush, N., Butler, L., Hassey, K., Ferrel, B., Grant, M., Gue, D., Hind, P., Kreuer, J., Padilla, G., & Underwood, S. (1997). Quality of life and the cancer experience: The state of the knowledge. *Oncology Nursing Forum*, 24, 27-41.

Last Acts Task Force. (1998). National policy statements on end-of-life care: Precepts of palliative care. *Journal of Palliative Medicine*, 1(2), 109-112. ·

Murphy, P., & Price, D. (1995). ACT: Taking a positive approach to end-of-life care. *American Journal of Nursing*, 3, 42-43.

Robert Wood Johnson Foundation Last Acts. (1996). *Last Acts: A strategy for change.* Internet.

Robert Wood Johnson Foundation. (December 3rd, 1998). *A Peaceful Death Symposium*, University of North Carolina, Chapel Hill, NC.

Sheenhan, D., & W. Forman (1996). *Hospice and palliative care: Concepts and Practice.* Sudbury, Mass.: Jones & Bartlett Publishers.

SUPPORT Study Investigators. (1995). A controlled trial to improve care for seriously ill hospitalized patients. *Journal of the American Medical Association*, 274(20), 1591-1598.

Hospice vs. Palliative Care

Patrice O'Connor

SUMMARY. A greater interest in end of life care has been emerging in the United States. A description of the evolution of hospice and palliative care is reviewed with issues such as studies and reports on the care of the dying, physician assisted suicide, medical education, the author's two hospital audit surveys and discussion of the challenges that face both hospice and palliative care. *[Article copies available for a fee from The Haworth Document Delivery Service: 1-800-342-9678. E-mail address: getinfo@haworthpressinc.com <Website: http://www.haworthpressinc.com>]*

KEYWORDS. Hospice, palliative care, palliative care initiatives, hospice/palliative care studies, palliative care demonstration projects, end-of-life care, end-of-life decision making

What people needed most when they are dying is relief from distressing symptoms of disease, security of a caring environment, sustained expert care and assurance that they and their families will not be abandoned. (Wald 1974)

INTRODUCTION:
HISTORY OF HOSPICE IN THE UNITED STATES

It has been 25 years since the first hospices were started in the United States. The question that needs to be asked is are we any closer

---

[Haworth co-indexing entry note]: "Hospice vs. Palliative Care." O'Connor, Patrice. Co-published simultaneously in *The Hospice Journal* (The Haworth Press, Inc.) Vol. 14, No. 3/4, 1999, pp. 123-137; and: *The Hospice Heritage: Celebrating Our Future* (ed: Inge B. Corless and Zelda Foster) The Haworth Press, Inc., 1999, pp. 123-137. Single or multiple copies of this article are available for a fee from The Haworth Document Delivery Service [1-800-342-9678, 9:00 a.m. - 5:00 p.m. (EST). E-mail address: getinfo@haworthpressinc.com].

123

to fulfilling the mandate that Florence Wald, the founder of the Hospice Movement in the United States, has stated as her challenge to health care.

The history of hospice in the United States is different than in England. As a grassroots movement, an alternative to acute aggressive care, the Hospice Movement started outside the medical community with no government funding. The basic elements of hospice care were the same as those of St. Christopher's Hospice–patient and family as the unit of care, pain and symptom control, and team approach. The first two hospice programs were structurally different from the St. Christopher's Hospice model. The Connecticut Hospice started in 1974 was a home care based program while the St. Luke's Hospice in New York City, started in the same year, was a hospital based scattered bed model. Along with the different base location of service–home vs. hospital a study done of the first hospices, indicated that admission criteria from the beginning were different in these two models. The hospice home care model required a primary care giver to be identified and the hospice hospital model did not require a care giver (O'Connor, Kaplan 1987).

The first National Hospice Conference was held in Washington in 1978. Based on the interest and support generated from this conference, the Federal Hospice Study was inaugurated in 1980, to 26 selected hospice programs in order to understand the new concept of "Hospice" and the possible inclusion of federal funding. Before the evaluation of the federal demonstration programs was completed, however the Medicare Hospice Benefit was enacted in 1984, as a result of political pressures by hospice constituencies. The Federal Medicare Hospice Benefit basic requirements were *(1) core staff and volunteers, (2) six months prognosis certified by a physician (3) patient informed consent, (4) set capital expense–daily rate and (5) 80% of the patient time, on the average of all patients, while on the program to be spent at home.* During this same period, New York State had approved a demonstration project. One of the results of New York Study was that patients were averaging 30% of their length of stay in the hospital. Even with these results, New York chose to follow the requirement of the Federal Hospice Benefit which allows only 20% of the length of stay to be in the hospital (Hannan, O'Donnell, 1984).

As to the projected cost savings which prompted the Federal funding, in the last month of life in 1997, patients using hospice accrued costs averaging $3,069, compared to $4,071 for non-hospice users. For longer periods, however, hospice care may actually raise costs, by substituting paid custodial and palliative care for care-taking previously provided by friends and family at no cost (Kelly 1998).

Licensure and Accreditation following passage of the Hospice Benefit was developed by the Joint Commission on Accreditation of Hospitals. Today, 43 states have hospice licensure laws and two have pending legislation. The Federal Hospice Benefit regulations are the basis of almost all of this legislation. Given that the Federal Hospice regulations mandates that patients be at home 80% of the time, the Hospice Home care model has become established as the primary Hospice model in the United States.

PALLIATIVE CARE

There has been a greater interest from the medical community in response to end-of-life care. The medical community has adopted the terms palliative medicine and palliative care. *The Oxford Textbook of Palliative Medicine* defines palliative care as the treatment prescribed by the physician practicing palliative medicine (*Oxford Textbook* 1993). Webster's dictionary offers a few definitions of palliative–to ease without curing and to cover by excuses and apologies. (Webster 1997).

The use of the term palliative care has been increasing in the past five years in the United States. In Canada hospices have always been called palliative care. The concept of palliative medicine and palliative care appears to be more acceptable to the medical community than the term hospice. Some of the reasons for this change may be the restrictiveness of the hospice regulations, the perceived death sentence of the word "hospice," the empty beds in acute care hospitals, the support and continuity of care given by caregivers for patients and families, starting the care approach early in the disease process, and the desire of patients and families who want to stop aggressive treatment.

In observing programs that are calling themselves "palliative care" there are a number of differences that can be noted from the Hospice model. Some of these differences are lack of spiritual care, limited social work, no volunteers, absence of home care visits, no coordination with the primary physician at the time of discharge or follow up and no bereavement services.

One way that this change is being introduced into the medical community is through undergraduate medical education. A recent status report on palliative care by Billings and Block on undergraduate medical education was based on their evaluation of over 9,000 citations on palliative care related topics that were retrieved from Medline searches from 1980 to 1995 and from reviewing 14 palliative care journals published from 1985 to 1996. There were 310 articles that addressed medical education for end-of-life care: 180 were carefully examined. Results indicated that curricular offerings were not well integrated and little attention was given to home care, hospice and nursing homes. The review also indicated role models were few and students were not encouraged to examine their personal reactions to their clinical experiences (Billings, Block 1997).

Another method of influencing the medical community has been joint partnerships to effect change in clinical practice. One joint venture was the National Hospice Organization and Annenberg Center for Health Sciences sponsored educational program regarding the care and treatment of dying patients. The purpose was to help chief residents introduce end-of-life issues to residents in family practice, internal medicine, geriatrics, and to fellows in oncology (Hospice Management Advisor, July 1997).

An important development has been the Health Care Financing Administration announcement of the approval of a new diagnosis code for palliative care on Oct. 1, 1996. The new code will enable coders to review hospital charts to indicate that palliative care was delivered to a dying patient during a hospital stay. As a result HCFA analysts will be able to study the feasibility of creating a special diagnosis-related group (DRG) that allows payment for end-of-life care for people who die in hospital or require hospitalization for palliative care close to the end of their lives (Cassel, 1996). This project has been started with limited success as hospitals are fearful of lack of reimbursement for identifying these patients since at present only acute care is reimbursed.

Hospice includes elements of palliative care but not all palliative care includes all the elements of hospice care. One would hope that time will prove that it is palliative defined as to ease without curing that is the care provided and not the second definition of palliative that is to cover by excuses and apologies that is the care being given. This second definition uses the term "palliative care" to the detriment of the patient's care and concerns (Webster 1997).

STUDIES AND REPORTS

What has brought the medical community to direct its focus on end-of-life care have been some major studies and reports that have analyzed how terminal care is practiced. Most of these studies were physician authored which indicates that the medical community is taking a leadership role in investigating the care of the dying. These studies and reports are mentioned here in chronological order to show the progression of interest in end-of-life care that has occurred in a very short period of time.

1. Brown Study (1983)–Federal funded study of 26 hospice pilot projects that outlined for the first time the profile of patient characteristics, the type of services that were being offered, different locations of services delivery models and financial costs (Greer 1986).
2. New York State Demonstration Project (1983)–New York was one of the first states to sponsor a study of 13 hospices selected as pilot projects. The results identified a regional response of one state to the new concept of "hospice care" by analyzing location of service and cost reporting (Hannan, O'Donnell 1984).
3. Support Study (1989 to 1994)–A study in an effort to achieve a clearer understanding of the character of dying in the American Hospital. This $28 million dollar project enrolled over 9,000 patients suffering from life-threatening illness in five United States teaching hospitals over a four-year period. The study demonstrated that physicians did not routinely query their patients about end-of-life decisions, and that they did not respond to interventions that had been designed to increase the frequency with which these discussions were made (Lynn 1995). Due to the negative outcome of the study's intervention, the Hastings Center published a special supplement that analyzed areas of medical education, ethics, and cultural differences which assisted in understanding what may be some of the reasons for the negative findings (Hastings Center 1995).

4. Solomon Study (1993) found that many physicians and nurses were disturbed by the degree to which technological solutions influence care during the final days of a terminal illness (Solomon 1993).

5. Project Death in America (1994) has sponsored projects and scholars to understand and transform the culture and experience of dying in the United States. Projects included initiatives in research, scholarship, the humanities, and the arts to foster innovations in the provision of care, public education, professional education, and public policy (PDIA 1996).

6. United Hospital Fund of New York Palliative Care Initiative (1996) provided grant support to 12 New York City hospitals to gather information about end-of-life care in their hospitals and to explore ways to improve this care. Five hospitals were selected to received funding for a two-year period to develop these projects (United Hospital Fund 1997).

7. Coalition for Compassionate Care Initiative (1995), composed of five large, integrated Catholic Health Care Systems and the Catholic Health Association, has been studying end-of-life care and developing its own model of comprehensive community based care (Hospice Management Advisor, July 1997).

8. American Board of Internal Medicine (1996) has produced a monograph on "Caring For the Dying" which includes identification and promotion of physician competency, as part of the American Board of Internal Medicine's End-of-Life Patient Care Project (ABIM 1996).

9. Robert Wood Johnson Foundation (1997) established a $12 million dollar initiative called "Promoting Excellence in End-of-Life Care" which aims to foster long-term changes in health care institutions that will improve end of life for the dying. Letters of intent were due Sept. 1997, 695 were received, 56 were asked to complete the Grant requests (Hospice Forum 1997).

10. Medicaring Project (1997) would enable patients to receive the kind of comfort hospice provides without giving up their right to curative treatment. The Health Care Financing Administration is considering the idea and some pilot projects are being planned to explore implementation issues such as service mix, eligibility, reimbursement levels, and Medicare waivers. Services could be similar to hospice, but extended out for a longer

period of time and thus would be less intensive and potentially more costly then the hospice current service package. Medicaring would be an opportunity to offer additional services in a different manner for patients with chronic heart and lung diseases or dementia (Hospice Management Advisor, Sept. 1997).

11. American College of Physicians (1997) has organized an End-of-Life Care Panel that is developing a set of state of the art reviews and resource material on end-of-life care (Hospice Management Advisor, Dec. 1997).

12. Institute of Medicine (1997)–the National Academy of Sciences has produced a report, "Approaching Death: Improving Care At the End-of-Life" (Cassel 1997).

13. American Medical Association (1997) has adopted two initiatives to improve end-of-life care, including projects focusing on education of physicians and patients and on improved effectiveness of "advance directives" (Hospice Management Advisor, Feb. 1997).

14. Last Acts (1997) is a broadly based coalition representing 72 organizations interested in improving the health care for the dying and was developed in direct response to the SUPPORT Study. This $1.7 million dollar project has as its primary goals to improve communication and decision making around end-of-life care, change how health care institutions treat dying patients, and influence broader cultural attitudes towards death (Hospice Management Advisor, Feb., 1997).

15. National Hospice Organization Hospice Benefit/End-of-Life Care Committee (1997) has as its charge the examination of the assumptions on which the Medicare Hospice Benefit rests, including strength, obstacles, access, functioning, structure and financing. The major task is to define some of the barriers to access–perceived or real–and look at characteristics of the Hospice of the future that will overcome these barriers (Hospice Letter 1997).

16. Time Tool Kit of Instruments to Measure End-of-Life Care (1997) has established a plan for filling in the blanks, for assembling a consensus among providers on outcomes,standards and practice guidelines in end-of-life care and for disseminating the results. The hope is to develop valid, clinically meaningful and manageable measures of quality that would apply to all settings

for end-of-life care, including hospice (Hospice Management Advisor, July 1997).

17. Memorial Study on Assisted Suicide (1997) reported that professional attitudes towards assisted suicide are influenced by diverse personal attributes, among which maybe competence in symptom management, burn out, and level of religious belief (Portenoy 1997).

18. ABCD (1998)–Americans for Better Care for the Dying is a new advocacy organization, a nonprofit organization dedicated to social, professional, and policy reform. There is a $50.00 membership fee used for financing activities with the purpose of demanding quality of care for the seriously ill, answering media inquiries, and drafting informed policy (Hospice Management Advisor, July 1997).

19. Gallup International Institute Survey (1998) found that most Americans long for spiritual support at the end-of-life. Fifty percent consider prayer important during that time and nearly as many as 44% would like to receive counseling to reach spiritual peace as they are dying (NHO Newsline 1998).

Hospice has been a beacon shedding light on the issues and concerns of the dying patients and families. It is estimated that 450,000 individuals used hospices in 1996 but this is less than 20% of all dying patients who could have qualified for the service. Who is giving the care to the other 80% of patients?

As one reflects on the above studies and reports, it becomes evident that the practice of the care of the dying has been receiving a great deal of attention from the medical community but the question remains as to how to change clinical practice to meet the identified concerns and needs.

TWO HOSPITAL SURVEYS

Just how does improved practice in the end-of-life care get translated to health care professional in the hospital setting? Two hospital surveys were conducted at medical centers in New York City. Each audit reviewed documentation and interviewed health care professionals who had dealt with the dying and death. The findings of both studies showed that staff were not educationally prepared or emotionally supported around the issues involved in care of the dying.

In the acute care setting there is a difference between death and dying. During a review of the medical record, it became evident that there were different types of death and dying that occur in the hospital setting–emergency room deaths, long term deaths such as those from cancer and AIDS, sudden deaths, deaths in the Intensive Care Units, and perinatal or neonatal deaths. Each of these was a death but the circumstances of the dying and the time frame and events leading to the death were very different. Yet it was expected that medical staff would response to these distinctions with little or no education or emotional support.

In both surveys, the medical record contained little documentation on interactions with patient and family concerning questions of what was death with dignity, when and where does it occur and who was involved in the decision-making process. The results of both studies indicated that there was no formal education in issues of dying and death in the medical setting, and no role modeling in clinical practice. The concerns expressed by the interns and residents included a fear of legal issues in decision making, and uncertainty of policy and procedures around end-of-life directives.

The nurses indicated they had received formal education in end-of-life care in both the undergraduate and graduate level. The concerns of the nurses in both studies were:

1. undermedication for pain even when pain concerns had been discussed with doctors.
2. lack of information on just what the patient and family had been told concerning the diagnosis and prognosis.
3. understaffing.
4. lack of support systems when staff experienced multiple deaths.

There are 103 medical schools and only one, the St. Louis University Medical School, has a required course with a curriculum in the care of the dying. Fifteen medical schools have an elective of one week on end-of-life care and the other medical schools stated they integrated the subject of caring for the dying patient and family into the education in general medicine. Most nursing curricula have a course on the death and dying. With the emerging role of nurse practitioner, it would be hoped that the nursing issues of end-of-life care will be addressed.

Of all the deaths in America, 80% of persons die in a health related institution (Hospice Management Advisor, July 1997). Support in the way of formal interdisciplinary in-service education is needed in order to enable staff to give quality care to both the patients and families.

PHYSICIAN-ASSISTED SUICIDE

One of the major questions facing those of the medical community who are involved in end-of-life care is physician assisted suicide. In this period of high-tech/medical treatment, and fear of intractable pain, and loss of physical and mental faculties, the issue of quality of life for patients is being reexamined. Regrettably, the debate is mostly centered in the legal arena. The Supreme Court has ruled that the matter of physician-assisted suicide should be settled at the state level (Quinn 1997). Oregon has passed legislation in 1994 and again in 1997 for physician-assisted suicide. Since September 1998, 10 patients were approved for physician-assisted suicide under the Oregon guidelines and 8 were assisted in their deaths.

The Attorney General of New York State has created a commission with the aim of studying the legal, social, educational and other barriers that prevent physicians from providing adequate care to patients in life's final stages (Hospice Management Advisor, Sept. 1997). Promoting alternatives to suffering or suicide for the dying will be major focus of this commission.

During the recent elections, the State of Michigan rejected legislation to approve physician-assisted suicide. This defeat was in part accomplished by the strong opposition of a consortium of groups composed of religious and pro-life groups. There are 35 states that expressly prohibit this practice and nine more states that would consider legislation but were waiting to see the results of the Michigan experience (*New York Times*, Nov. 12, 1998). Some of the hospice responses to physician-assisted suicide legislation have been like that of the Benton Hospice Services, Inc. of Oregon that developed a philosophy, policy and procedures for addressing this situation. They have stated that they will not abandon dying patients and families but will not actively participate in physician-assisted suicide (Hospice Management Advisor, July 1997).

The Connecticut Hospice has been instrumental in helping the state of Connecticut to offer an official notice of desire for hospice called physician-assisted living. The physician-assisted living initiative establishes a patient's bill of rights, under which individuals may complete this advance directive to indicate their desire for a dignified death and palliative care (Califano 1998).

Physician and ethicist Sulmasy states "assisted suicide and euthanasia are, in themselves, morally problematic activities for the medical profession. Yet even persons so persuaded will at least recognize that legalizing euthanasia and assisted suicide at the time of intense pressures to control the cost of health care is unwise, it is like alcohol and gasoline, managed care and managed death do not mix" (Sulmasy 1995). Both hospice and palliative care are confronting this issue, which may be one of the essential differences between the two that will emerge in the future. The type of patients who will seek out palliative care and may be interested in physician assisted suicide may not be terminally ill but those who question their quality of life due to some chronic illness.

CROSSROADS

At the time hospice was being developed in the United States, in the 1970s the focus of decision-making was the physician and patient, the appropriateness of care was clinical appropriateness and desirability, the economics of health care was viewed as abundant and financial arrangement was fee for service, the focus of care was the interest of the individual patient and the basis of standards was professional judgment. The picture has completely changed today. The focus of decision-making is third party payers and legislation, and the meaning of appropriateness is cost-worthiness (appropriate within limited resources). The financial arrangement is managed care, the normative focus is the interest of all patients in resource availability and the interest of the stockholders and the basis of standards is evidence and cost (Sharpe, 1997). Each new change develops within a climate that is accepting of the idea. Even though hospice started outside the medical community, it was the environment of how health care was delivered that enabled hospice to start and is now its most challenging factor in making it change or fade away.

When hospices first started they were non-profit organizations. The focus of financial management has changed in that there are for-profit hospices that are offering stock on Wall Street (Hospice Management Advisor, July 1997). At the present time, the funding for palliative care is under traditional health care reimbursement until such time as the Federal Government decides to enact a diagnosis related groups reimbursement schedule for palliative care.

Within the professional organizations of the health care groups involved in end-of-life care, there have been changes. The American Academy of Hospice Physicians is now the American Academy of Hospice and Palliative Medicine, and the Hospice Nursing Association is the Hospice and Palliative Nurse's Association. The name changes indicate the awareness of the health care professional that in order to insure the principles of hospice care are maintained in health care delivery, they needed to reach out to a wider group of health care professionals. There are now certifications granted by both professional organizations.

One of the results of the SUPPORT Study indicated that 58% of the patients were not interested in discussing their preference for CPR (Lynn 1997) and yet a requirement for admission to hospice is a signed informed consent by the patient. This would indicate again the reluctance to discuss issues around end-of-life decision making and result in patients staying within a system of health care delivery which has no such requirements. This limits the number of patients who recognize their eligibility to receive hospice care and consequently do not enter the program. In order to reach a broader population of patients, hospices are now serving patients in nursing homes. In New York State, 42 hospices are involved in giving hospice care to patients and support to staff within 453 nursing homes (Brooks 1997).

If one can imagine hospice as a boat in the storm of a changing health care ocean, it is difficult to predict what the future will hold. Some of the areas that will have to be addressed are financial pressures, organizations entering into a variety of new relationships with managed care organizations, home health agencies, and hospitals. Finally, there are cultural and social challenges as Americans struggle with legal and moral issues of death and dying. Hospices have been successful in addressing the needs of middle class white elderly persons with cancer who have families. However, there is a need to provide better access to care within diverse settings and for diverse populations. Many patients find that the term "hospice" depressing and wish to continue the dance of denial. In this age of uncertainty in health care, financial pressures have other providers hold on to their own hospice appropriate patients to maximize their own income.

Health care today is controlled by finances (government, insurance, health management organization, managed care) and legal controls (Quinlan Case, Cruzan Case, Physician Assisted Suicide Legislation in Oregon State (Gostin 1997)). Hospice needs to develop resources to meet the needs of patients that fall outside the range of reimbursed service. Hospice can no longer be an isolated self-contained service delivery system.

Recently, the U.S. Department of Health and Human Services' Office of Inspector General as part of Operation Restore Trust alleged that hospices have admitted thousands of ineligible patients. While highly respected and successful in its mission, the Medicare hospice program has experienced a substantial number of ineligible enrollments, according to the report. This situation emphasizes the difficulty for hospice programs of defining a terminal prognosis. The SUPPORT Study has emphasized the difficulties in making a terminal prognosis by stating that neither attending physician nor computerized statistical models were able to predict prognoses with more than 50% accuracy (Lynn, 1995).

Patients preferring to wait until much later before accepting a hospice referral have contributed to a shortened length of stay for hospice programs. The National Hospice Organization Fact Sheet for 1996 indicates that the typical hospice is non-profit and operates with a patient census between 10 and 100 (Hospice Letter 1997). How they will be able to survive in this changing health care delivery system is not clear.

Palliative care is still in the early stages of development in United States. Palliative medicine has been a specialty in England and Canada for some time. The pressures on the medical community for better end-of-life care has challenged physicians to practice palliative medicine which will then be translated into palliative care by an interdisciplinary team.

CONCLUSION

The purpose of this paper is to show the early history of hospice and the development of an interest in palliative care in the medical community which was not present at the beginning of the Hospice movement in United States. Since 80% of all deaths occur in a health-related institution and medical education and training also occurs in the same inpatients settings, the development of principles of care of the dying means the encouragement of palliative care. But if palliative care does not contain all basic elements of hospice care such as developing and monitoring of symptom control, patient and family support, home care services, bereavement services, research and evaluation, education and training, then we have severely limited its contribution to the dying patients, family and health care professionals. It is not a matter of either/or but a blend of both that is needed to met the needs of end-of-life care.

Are we any closer to fulfilling the mandate and challenge that Wald offered at the beginning of hospice development in the United States? The answer is yes but in different forms based on the ever-evolving health care delivery system and education of health care professionals in the United States. The future looks bright because some of the physicians leading the development of palliative care have been hospice physicians who are attempting to bring the strength of both services to the common goal of good patient care.

REFERENCES

American Board of Internal Medicine. (1996). *Care for the Dying, Identification and Promotion of Physician Competency.* Philadelphia, p. 1-100.

Billings, J.A.; Block, S. (1997). Palliative Care in Undergraduate Medical Education: Status Report and Future Direction. *Journal of the American Medical Association,* 278(9):733-738.

Brooks, S. (1997). Of Hope and Hospice. *Contemporary Long Term Care,* Jul:36-62.

Califano, J. (1998). Physician-Assisted Living. *America,* 14:10-12.

Cassel, C. (1997). *Approaching Death–Improving Care at the End of Life.* National Academy of Science, National Academy Press.

Cassel, C.; Vladeck, B. (1996). ICD-9 Code for Palliative or Terminal Care. *New England Journal of Medicine,* 335(16):1232-1233.

Doyle, D.; Hanks, G.; Mac Donald, N. (1993). *Oxford Textbook of Palliative Medicine.* Oxford Medical Pub, United Kingdom (2nd Edition).

Gallup International Institute. (1998). Spiritual Support. *National Hospice Organization Newsletter* Jan. 1:7.

Gostin, L. (1997). Health Law and Ethics, Deciding Life and Death in the Court Room. *Journal of the American Medical Association,* 278, (18):1523-1528.

Greer, D.; Mor, V.; Morris, J.; Sherwood, S.; Kidder, D.; Birnbaum, H. (1986). An Alternative in Terminal Care: Results of the National Hospice Study. *Journal of Chronic Diseases,* 39(1):9-26.

Hannan, E.L.; O'Donnell, J.F. (1984). An Evaluation of Hospices in the New York State Hospice Demonstration Program. *Inquiry,* 21: 338-348.

Hastings Center Report; Special Supplement. (1995). *Dying Well in the Hospital,* 25(6):S1-S36.

Hospice Letter. (1997). New Grant Program Focuses on Improving Care For the Dying. *Hospice Letter,* 19(1):8-9.

Hospice Management Advisor. (1997). Coalition for Compassionate Care. *Instinctive American Health Consultants,* 1(7):78.

Hospice Management Advisor. (1997). Medicaring Project. *American Health Consultants,* 1(9):109-110.

Hospice Management Advisor. (1997). American College Of Physicians–End of Life Care. *American Health Consultants,* 1(12):134-136.

Hospice Management Advisor. (1997). Advance Directives. *American Health Consultants,* 1(2):16.

Hospice Management Advisor. (1997). Last Acts. *American Health Consultants.* 1(2):18.

Hospice Management Advisor. (1997). Time Tool Kit. *American Health Consultants.* 1(7):72-73.

Hospice Management Advisor. (1997). Americans for Better Care for the Dying. *American Health Consultants,* 1(7):73-74.

Hospice Management Advisor. (1997). Benton Hospice Services. *American Health Consultants,* 1(7):75-76.

Kelly, A.; Gabel, J.; Hurst, K. (1998) The Truth About Hospice. *Business and Health,* 16(9):67-68.

Lynn, J.; Teno, J.; Harrell, F.M. (1995). A Controlled Trial to Improve Care for Seriously Ill Hospitalized Patients. *Journal of the American Medical Association* 274(20):1591-8.

Lynn, J. (1997) Perceptions by family members of the Dying Experience of Older and Seriously Ill Patients. *Annals of Internal Medicine* 126 (2):97-106.

National Hospice Organization. (1997). Hospice Benefit/End of Life Care Committee Legislative Alert. *Hospice Letter,* 19(5):1-5.

New York Times, Nov. 12, 1998:1-12.

O'Connor, P.; Kaplan, M. (1987). The Effects of Medicare Regulations, an Access to Hospice Care: Requirements for Primary Care Persons in American Hospices. *American Journal of Hospice Care* Nov/Dec:34-42.

Portenoy, R, (1997). Determinants of the Willingness to Endorse Assisted Suicide. *Psychosomatic* 38:277-287.

Project Death in America. (1996). *PDIA Newsletter,* Open Society Institute. 1:1.

Quinn, T. (1997). Health, Law and Ethics, Palliative Options of Last Resort. *Journal of the American Medical Association,* 278(23):2099-2104.

Sharpe, V. (1997). The Politics, Economics, and Ethics of "Appropriateness." *Kennedy Institute of Ethics Journal,* 7(4):337-343.

Solomon, M. (1993). Decisions near the end of life: Professional views on life-sustaining treatments. *American Journal of Public Health,* 83(1):14-25.

Sulmasy, D. (1995). Managed Care and Managed Death. *Archives of Internal Medicine,* 155(3):133-136.

United Hospital Fund. (1997) Palliative Care Initiative. *Blueprint,* Spring:6.

Wald, F.; Foster, Z. Wald, H. (1980). The Hospice Movement As A Health Care Reform. *Nursing Outlook. March*:134-137.

Webster's Dictionary (1997): 503.

The NHO
Medical Guidelines for Non-Cancer Disease
and Local Medical Review Policy:
Hospice Access for Patients with Diseases
Other Than Cancer

Brad Stuart

SUMMARY. For much of its history, hospice focused on problems related to malignant disease. Recently, however, non-cancer diagnoses such as congestive heart failure, emphysema and Alzheimer's disease have comprised an increasing proportion of hospice referrals. This paper details criteria published by NHO and adopted by the US Health Care Financing Administration for hospice eligibility for common non-cancer diagnoses. A provisional list of domains for documenting "evidence of rapid decline," by which patients with advanced disease who do not meet criteria can still be certified for the Medicare Hospice Benefit, is also outlined. *[Article copies available for a fee from The Haworth Document Delivery Service: 1-800-342-9678. E-mail address: getinfo@haworthpressinc.com <Website: http://www.haworthpressinc.com>]*

KEYWORDS. Non-cancer disease, NHO guidelines, LMRP, rapid decline

INTRODUCTION

The first US hospice program opened in 1974, funded by a three-year grant from the National Cancer Institute. Ten years later, when

---

[Haworth co-indexing entry note]: "The NHO *Medical Guidelines for Non-Cancer Disease* and Local Medical Review Policy: Hospice Access for Patients with Diseases Other Than Cancer." Stuart, Brad. Co-published simultaneously in *The Hospice Journal* (The Haworth Press, Inc.) Vol. 14, No. 3/4, 1999, pp. 139-154; and: *The Hospice Heritage: Celebrating Our Future* (ed: Inge B. Corless and Zelda Foster) The Haworth Press, Inc., 1999, pp. 139-154. Single or multiple copies of this article are available for a fee from The Haworth Document Delivery Service [1-800-342-9678, 9:00 a.m. - 5:00 p.m. (EST). E-mail address: getinfo@haworthpressinc.com].

Congress passed legislation creating the Medicare Benefit, hospice care was focused mainly on relieving the pain and suffering associated with malignant disease. Today, hospice's expertise in management of the medical, psychosocial and spiritual aspects of terminal cancer is widely acknowledged.

But over the quarter century since its inception, hospice's role has broadened. Today non-cancer diagnoses like congestive heart failure (CHF) and chronic obstructive pulmonary disease (COPD) account for an ever-larger proportion of hospice enrollments. This growth has challenged hospice and the US Health Care Financing Administration (HCFA) to create workable systems for hospice enrollment, Medicare Benefit certification and reimbursement.

REIMBURSEMENT EFFECTS ON ELIGIBILITY

Medicare Hospice Benefit legislation legitimized end-of-life care, making hospice equivalent to other reimbursable medical services. For the first time, care of the dying was institutionalized and publicly supported. However, the new law also placed restrictions on patient eligibility for hospice unlike any other segment of the US health care system. Other Medicare-covered services, even those financed under specialized benefits, i.e., dialysis for End-Stage Renal Disease (ESRD), were provided to patients throughout the course of illness. Eligibility for hospice patients, on the other hand, was restricted to those with "a life expectancy of six months or less, assuming the disease runs its normal course."

As long as hospice enrolled predominantly cancer patients, this "six-month rule" did not pose much of a problem, since the "normal course" of cancer is characterized by inexorable and obvious clinical decline for several months prior to death. However, from the mid-1980s onward, patients with non-cancer diagnoses comprised an increasing proportion of hospice referrals. This was due to a number of factors including the aging of the US population with an attendant increase in prevalence of chronic disease, growing hospice expertise in management of non-pain symptoms such as dyspnea and agitation, significant capital formation in a number of successful hospice programs linked to effective physician education and targeted marketing for new kinds of referrals, declines in traditional fee-for-service reimbursement to physicians and hospitals making aggressive treatment of end-stage disease less profitable, and a slowly-growing awareness among physicians and in the culture at large that a well-managed death was an appropriate and positive therapeutic goal.

Continued growth of hospice into the non-cancer arena met with resistance from HCFA in the mid-1990s. Hospice had always viewed late referrals as a major problem, because enrollment extremely late in the disease process resulted in short patient stays with little time for development of relationships critical to hospice's effectiveness. A landmark study in 1995 documented that up to fifteen percent of new hospice enrollees died within a week of admission.[1]

However, the study also showed that about fifteen percent of patients survived longer than six months. These long-stay patients were defined by HCFA as non-terminal and therefore as ineligible for the Medicare Hospice Benefit. This judgment was reinforced as the US Office of the Inspector General's "Operation Restore Trust" attempted to force certain large hospice programs to refund millions of Medicare Benefit dollars paid for patients surviving beyond 210 days, alleging this revenue was obtained through "fraud and abuse" rather than prognostic uncertainty. Although a few of these patients were victims of breast or prostate cancer, the majority had primary diagnoses of CHF, COPD and Alzheimer's disease.

THE CHALLENGE OF NON-CANCER DISEASE

Traditionally, US physicians have not felt comfortable with labeling patients with far-advanced CHF, COPD, Alzheimer's and other non-cancer diseases as "terminal," unlike those with end-stage cancer. Exacerbations of non-cancer disease, regardless of severity, have been considered "treatable" or even "curable" until death finally defeats the efforts of the clinician. Contributing to this attitude is the fact that endotracheal intubation and mechanical ventilation can keep patients with end-stage CHF and COPD technically alive until physiologic reserve is completely exhausted.

Physicians also have been reluctant to refer patients to hospice because of the prognostic uncertainty inherent in non-cancer disease. Even when aggressive measures give way to supportive treatment, patients can live for long periods at very low levels of function. With threats of monetary penalties for physicians referring "inappropriate" patients to hospice, later referrals and diminished lengths of stay have become commonplace.

Prognostic uncertainty in non-cancer patients is a serious problem for hospice. In contrast to patients with advanced cancer, who tend to follow a relatively relentless and therefore predictable downhill course over the last few months of life, those with non-cancer diagnoses tend to remain clinically stable for long periods, then suffer unpredictable exacerbations.[2] These downturns may or may not respond to treatment. Six-month prognosis is therefore extremely difficult to determine in most cases. In fact, prognosis in non-cancer patients is very difficult to determine even in seriously-ill hospitalized patients,[3] whose physicians have easy access to far more data than is usually available to hospice at the time of admission.

In addition, hospice care can stabilize patients with non-cancer disease, thereby prolonging life. This occurs more commonly in non-cancer illness than in cancer, since the medications used for palliation of non-cancer symptoms are frequently the same ones used for active disease-modifying treatment. Whereas in end-stage cancer active chemotherapy and radiation eventually give way to pain relief with opioids, in CHF palliation of dyspnea is best achieved through judicious administration of opioids along with diuretics and angiotensin-converting enzyme (ACE) inhibitors, which have been shown to lengthen life significantly in many studies.

THE NHO GUIDELINES FOR NON-CANCER DISEASE

In 1994, under the guidance of the National Hospice Organization (NHO), several hospice medical directors began work on a set of guidelines for hospices to use in deciding whether to certify patients for the Medicare Benefit. The First Edition of NHO's *Medical Guidelines for Determining Prognosis in Selected Non-Cancer Diseases*[4] was published in 1995, including CHF, COPD and Alzheimer's disease. The Second Edition of the *Medical Guidelines*[5] was published the next year, with additional criteria for AIDS, liver and renal disease, stroke and coma and amyotrophic lateral sclerosis (ALS).

Contrary to their title, the *Medical Guidelines* do not literally "predict prognosis." Because they are based on a synthesis of available literature rather than quantitative studies in hospice populations with six-month survival as a measured outcome, they are neither sensitive nor specific in individual cases. Even with research to optimize their predictive validity, it is questionable whether the *Medical Guidelines* or any other set of criteria simple enough to be applied in clinical situations will ever predict six-month life expectancy. In fact, experienced investigators have stated that prognosis of mortality will probably never be an exact science.[6]

Nevertheless, shortly after their publication the *Medical Guidelines* were adapted by HCFA into Local Medical Review Policy (LMRP) as standards for hospice reimbursement, despite protests by NHO, the American Academy of Hospice and Palliative Medicine and others. The five Medicare Fiscal Intermediaries (FI's) have now created their own LMRP based on the HCFA policies. Considerable effort by hospice and FI Medical Directors over the past two years has been devoted to creating a workable system that does not deny access to hospice-appropriate patients, yet provides the FI's with valid criteria to prevent true fraud and abuse.

The following is a brief description of major guidelines for the main non-cancer diagnoses seen in hospice. For convenience, they are presented as they have evolved in LMRP discussions, in the form adopted recently by Blue Cross of California, the West Coast FI. These criteria are meant to be used for certifying patients for the Medicare Hospice Benefit. They are not portrayed as definitions of hospice appropriateness, since a hospice may choose to admit a patient and provide services outside the Benefit, supported for instance by community contributions.

It is critical to understand that patients who appear to be within six months of death but fall outside these criteria may still be appropriate for hospice enrollment and Medicare Benefit certification. LMRP provide for this by allowing hospices to document "evidence of rapid decline" outside LMRP criteria. This documentation is also useful when considering whether to certify patients for subsequent Benefit periods after the first. Domains for documentation of clinical decline will be discussed further below.

HEART DISEASE

Patients with advanced CHF are considered appropriate for hospice if they are (1) *symptomatic at rest* (New York Heart Association Class IV) and (2) already *optimally treated with diuretics and vasodilators*.

The latter medications are usually in the ACE-inhibitor category. If referred patients are not on these medications, the attending physician should be asked why not, because even very advanced CHF patients may benefit significantly both symptomatically and in terms of life expectancy. Fears of worsening renal insufficiency or hypotension with the use of ACE inhibitors may be unfounded even in Class IV heart failure.[7] If these medications have not been considered by the physician, the patient may not be hospice-appropriate unless he or she refuses them. Hospice staff who are experienced in management of volume status, blood pressure and electrolytes may choose, in collaboration with physicians, to titrate dosages of diuretics and ACE inhibitors to control CHF symptoms, although discharge may be necessary if patients stabilize or improve.

CHF patients are usually appropriate for hospice when they have failed trials of intravenous inotropics such as dobutamine or milrinone. Elderly patients with intractable angina who are not candidates for coronary revascularization may also be hospice candidates when they no longer respond well to nitrates, beta- and calcium-channel blockers and other appropriate medications, although these may still be useful along with morphine in relieving cardiac pain.

Other factors supporting hospice eligibility are listed in the *Medical Guidelines* or LMRP.

Even though prognosis is difficult in CHF, with experience referring physicians and hospice staff can learn to select those patients who are "terminal." In a recent series of forty CHF patients enrolled in hospice at one of the branches of our agency, only five survived longer than six months. Median survival of the remaining cohort was about two months. Post-death surveys revealed high levels of patient, family and physician satisfaction.[8]

PULMONARY DISEASE

Prognosis is challenging in end-stage lung disease because most patients die of sudden and unpredictable exacerbations rather than chronic decline. Many exacerbations occur in the fall and winter when upper respiratory infections are prevalent.

These patients usually have end-stage obstructive disease, i.e., emphysema or chronic bronchitis, with severe *fixed* obstruction to expiration. It is important to carefully evaluate patients with *reversible* obstructive disease, i.e., asthma, because those patients who respond to bronchodilators probably have a better prognosis. Some patients with *restrictive* disease, e.g., pulmonary fibrosis, may also be eligible.

Pulmonary patients are hospice-appropriate if they have (1) *severe* and (2) *progressive* lung disease. They should also have either (3) *hypoxemia OR* (4) *hypercapnia*.

Severe pulmonary disease, like heart disease, produces disabling symptoms at rest or with minimal exertion, and results in diminished functional capacity, i.e., bed-to-chair existence. If pulmonary function tests are available, a post-bronchodilator Forced Expiratory Volume in One Second (FEV1) of less than thirty percent of the predicted value is helpful, but not required. Note that performance this poor implies unresponsiveness to bronchodilators by definition.

Progressive disease is evidenced by increasing Emergency Department visits (two in prior six months) or hospitalizations (one in prior year) for pulmonary infections or respiratory failure. Patients are more likely to be within six months of death if they have undergone intubation and mechanical ventilation, or at least continuous positive airway pressure ventilation during an exacerbation, especially if they state they do not want to undergo these procedures again.

Hypoxemia is defined as having a pO2 of less than or equal to 55 mm Hg on arterial blood gases (ABG), or oxygen saturation (SaO2) of less than or equal to 88% on oximetry. These values should be obtained on room air, off supplemental oxygen. *Hypercapnia* is evidenced by a pCO2 of greater than or equal to 50 mm Hg on ABG. Note that oximetry, which can be performed at the bedside in the patient's home, is all that is required. ABG values, however, may often be obtained from Emergency visits or recent hospitalizations.

Other helpful information includes evidence of *cor pulmonale,* i.e., right heart failure due to lung disease, not CHF or valvular disease; *weight loss* of greater than 10% in 6 months; and *resting tachycardia* of greater than one hundred beats per minute. This last item is a physical finding that is easily assessed at the bedside.

DEMENTIA

As dementia becomes more severe, mortality rises, but it is very hard to predict when patients are within six months of dying because the dementing process is not the primary cause of death. Dementia patients die from secondary medical complications, not from the dementia itself. Conversely, some patients are so demented they score zero on mental status tests, yet live for years with meticulous care.

Hospice criteria for dementia include: (1) dementia of sufficient *severity* and (2) the first occurrence of *medical complications.*

Dementia *severity* qualifies for hospice when the patient has passed Stage 7-C of the Functional Assessment Staging (FAST) scale. Briefly, these patients have lost the ability to ambulate independently and carry on meaningful conversation. They also have lost the ability to carry out most or all Activities of Daily Living (ADLs) and are at least occasionally incontinent of urine and/or stool.

Medical complications herald significant downturns in most demented patients. Those most often seen include aspiration pneumonia, upper urinary tract infection often including sepsis, worsening multiple stage 3-4 decubiti, fever recurrent after a course of antibiotics or greater than ten percent weight loss over six months.

Because of prognostic uncertainty in advanced dementia, these criteria are somewhat restrictive. Many demented patients, particularly those with other comorbid conditions, may be clearly terminal and still not qualify. These patients should be admitted to hospice with clear documentation of comorbidities and evidence of rapid decline. They may then be discharged if they stabilize.

HIV DISEASE

With the advent of protease inhibitors, AIDS mortality has declined. However, not all patients respond to these agents, and many cannot or will not comply with demanding drug regimens.

Patients with HIV disease are considered hospice-appropriate if they have both:

- *CD4+ (T-cell) count* of less than or equal to 25 and
- *Viral load* of greater than or equal to 100,000 copies/ml.

In addition, they should have a *decreased functional status* corresponding to less than or equal to 50 on the Karnofsky Performance Status (KPS) scale, as well as at least one of the following AIDS-related conditions:

- Central nervous system or poorly responsive systemic lymphoma.

- Wasting: loss of more than thirty-three percent of lean body mass.
- Mycobacterium avium complex (MAC) bacteremia.
- Progressive multifocal leukoencephalopathy (PML).
- Refractory visceral Kaposi's sarcoma (KS).
- Renal failure in the absence of dialysis.
- Refractory cryptosporidium infection.
- Refractory toxoplasmosis.

Other factors supporting hospice eligibility are listed in the Medical Guidelines and LMRP.

LIVER DISEASE

Cirrhosis is the final common pathway for most of the conditions that cause liver cell death of sufficient degree to overwhelm the liver's considerable capacity for regeneration. The criteria below thus refer mainly to end-stage cirrhosis, although other diagnoses such as sclerosing cholangitis may also be appropriate. Patients awaiting liver transplant are hospice-eligible but should be taken off the Medicare Benefit through revocation or discharge if a donor organ becomes available. As with other conditions, cirrhotic patients who appear terminal but whose laboratory data do not qualify them can still be enrolled if comorbidities and evidence of rapid decline can be documented.

Patients are hospice-appropriate when their *laboratory values* include both:

- *Prothrombin time* elevated more than five seconds over control, or International Normalized Ratio (*INR*) greater than 1.5, and
- Serum *albumin* less than 2.5.

In addition, the patient should have one or more of the following *medical conditions associated with advanced liver failure*:

- Ascites despite diuretics.
- Episode of spontaneous bacterial peritonitis.
- Hepatorenal syndrome.
- Hepatic encephalopathy despite lactulose.
- Recurrent bleeding esophageal varices despite therapy.

Other factors supporting hospice eligibility are listed in the Medical Guidelines or LMRP.

RENAL DISEASE

Every patient discontinuing renal dialysis for end-stage renal disease (ESRD) should be considered for hospice. All anuric post-dialysis patients die within days, but those who produce even small amounts of urine may have residual renal function that can enable them to live for weeks or, in rare cases, months. Six-month survival, of course, is extremely rare.

Laboratory criteria for hospice eligibility include:

- Serum *creatinine* greater than or equal to 8.0 mg/dl.
- *Creatinine clearance* less than or equal to 10 ml/min (15 ml/min. for diabetics).

To avoid collecting a twenty-four hour urine collection, creatinine clearance may be calculated according to the following formula:

$$\text{Creatinine Clearance} = \frac{(140 - \text{age in years})(\text{body weight in kilograms})}{72 \, (\text{serum creatinine in mg/dl})}$$

For women, multiply result by 0.85.

The same laboratory values apply for patients in *acute renal failure.* This condition may occur in the elderly as a result of sepsis, myocardial infarction or other insult, or in younger patients from massive trauma or other cause of circulatory collapse. These patients are often hospitalized, so if the patient is not dialyzed, inpatient hospice may be appropriate, or hospice services can be provided at home after discharge.

STROKE AND COMA

Patients who present in coma after cerebrovascular accident (CVA) rarely survive if the coma persists beyond three days, and thus are appropriate for hospice. Of course, post-CVA patients with complete dysphagia who do not receive feeding tubes are eligible as well. Caution should be exercised in evaluating patients immediately post CVA for hospice if they have stabilized or begun to improve neurologically, since further improvement is likely unless the area of infarction recurs or extends.

In the chronic phase after CVA, i.e., after the patient has progressed through convalescence or rehabilitation to a stable condition, criteria for hospice include either (1) post-stroke dementia equivalent to Stage 7-C of the FAST scale as detailed above under DEMENTIA, (2) poor functional status corresponding to a KPS of 40 or less, or (3) weight loss of ten percent over six months or less, or serum albumin less than 2.5.

Patients in coma are eligible for hospice if they show any three of the following four findings:

- Abnormal brain stem response.
- No response to verbal stimuli.
- No withdrawal to painful stimuli.
- Serum creatinine greater than 1.5 mg/dl.

The same medical complications listed under DEMENTIA also support, but are not necessary for, hospice eligibility. Diagnostic imaging findings that also support hospice appropriateness are listed in the *Medical Guidelines* and LMRP.

DETERMINING HOSPICE ELIGIBILITY FOR PATIENTS WHO DO NOT FIT LMRP CRITERIA

Research is now underway to determine the predictive validity of the *Medical Guidelines* and LMRP, and to include psychosocial and spiritual as well as medical variables. However, results will not be available for several years. Until then, hospice must make do with LMRP selection criteria, bearing in mind that they are not based on empirical data. Until these policies become evidence-based, they will probably not be either *sensitive* or *specific*–not sensitive, because they will disqualify certain patients who will die within six months, and not specific, because they will qualify others who will survive longer than six months.

Efforts to increase both sensitivity and specificity, characteristics of any set of selection criteria, are generally in opposition. That is, attempts to make criteria more specific can cause them to be less sensitive, and vice versa. In LMRP terms, "tightening up" eligibility criteria for hospice, i.e., requiring patients to be sicker in an attempt to increase specificity, might indeed result in fewer six-month survivors. However, fewer patients would be enrolled overall and more would die within six months without ever becoming eligible for hospice. The writers of the NHO *Medical Guidelines* and those who drafted LMRP therefore tried to strike a middle course between the extremes of sensitivity and specificity.

Until LMRP allow more accurate prediction of six-month life expectancy–assuming acceptable predictive validity is attainable–these problems must be confronted by providers of care. Since LMRP do not possess either specificity or sensitivity to allow hospice to predict six-month survival in advance, hospice must compensate on a concurrent basis. Unfortunate effects of LMRP non-specificity and insensitivity can both be avoided, although the means are not optimal scientifically, or from a patient care perspective.

Specificity is optimized when few patients are kept on the Benefit beyond six months, unless they are clearly declining. The only way to achieve this is to discharge patients who stabilize during the first or second Benefit periods. On further decline, these patients can be re-enrolled and certified for another Benefit period. Theoretically, with recent changes in the law abolishing the Third and Fourth Benefit periods and substituting an unlimited number of renewable sixty-day periods, discharges and readmissions can be readily accomplished. In practice, continuity of care suffers with this approach. Also, anecdotally many patients who are discharged because they appear stable under hospice care die shortly thereafter.

Sensitivity is of great concern to hospice, because it is synonymous with access to hospice services. Insensitive eligibility criteria deny hospice services to patients who will die within six months. In order to allow eligibility for patients who do not fit LMRP criteria but are apparently terminal, the policies provide for enrollment with documentation of "evidence of rapid decline."

EVIDENCE OF RAPID DECLINE

Medicare Medical Review personnel are trained to look for evidence of clinical decline in the hospice medical record to document eligibility. They seek clinical information, both from the referring physician's records sent by hospice and from the initial and subsequent evaluations by hospice staff, to differentiate the hospice patient's "terminal" course from that of chronic illness. Documentation is required of the *tangible medical reasons for enrollment*, rather than a description of care delivered, even though the latter information may be vital to remain in compliance with other regulations. This information is also useful to hospice staff to document whether patients should be certified for subsequent Benefit periods when the patient survives the first.

The clinical parameters shown in Table 1 have been useful in documenting clinical decline. Both objective and subjective elements are included, since individualized narrative information is needed to provide a detailed clinical picture to Medicare medical reviewers. The data may be gathered as a baseline on admission evaluation and, if the patient remains alive, again after two and five months to help with certification decisions for Benefit periods subsequent to the first. It

TABLE 1. Parameters for monitoring and documenting clinical decline.

History
Exam
Karnovsky score
Level of activity
Ambulation
ADL's
    Bathing
    Feeding
    Dressing
    Toileting
    Transferring
    Continence
    Urinary
    Fecal
Nutritional status
Weight
    Present
    6 months ago
Anthropometrics
    Triceps skin fold thickness
    Abdominal girth
    Mid-arm circumference
Mental status

may also be helpful on initial evaluation to ask about the status of each parameter one to three months previously to provide historical comparison.

Although many elements that may impact survival are gathered together here, not all of them apply to each case. "Anthropometric measurements," for instance, are useful for documenting decline in patients who cannot get out of bed to be weighed. This information is useful for patients with "Debility and Decline," i.e., no formal diagnosis, or those with Alzheimer's disease.

Table 2 provides sample data for a patient with CHF. Clinical find-

TABLE 2. Sample data for a patient with CHF.

History: Dyspnea with any exertion.
 Orthopnea: must prop up on 2 pillows to sleep.
 Paroxysmal nocturnal dyspnea 2-3 nights/wk.
Exam: JVD to 4 cm above clavicles.
 Rales to ½.
 3+ edema to knees.
Karnovsky score: 40
Level of activity: Chairbound, some bedrest.
Ambulation: with moderate assist.
ADLs:
 Bathing: shower chair with assist.
 Feeding: no problem.
 Dressing: no problem; bathrobe only.
 Toileting: assist to commode.
 Incontinence:
  Urinary: 1-2/wk.
  Fecal: no.
Nutritional status: poor; will not eat low-salt diet.
Weight:
 Present: 115 lb.
 6 months ago: 120 lb.
Anthropometrics:
 Triceps skinfold thickness:
 Abdominal girth:
 Mid-arm circumference:
Mental status: oriented; sometimes drowsy.
Other: Wants to lie in dark room alone last 2 weeks.
 Refuses meds 2-3x/wk.
 Refuses to go to see doctor last 1 month.

ings from both history and physical exam are emphasized, because they give a picture of disease severity and therefore some indication of survivability, although there is not a strict correlation between the two. Under "Other" may be listed further concise narrative that specifically describes how the patient is withdrawing or declining. Relevant psychosocial material that fleshes out the clinical picture may be documented here.

Because the goal of this documentation is to provide a unique picture of the patient's clinical status to a reviewer, the data is narrative in form. However, after review and revision, a list such as this could be standardized and used to gather programmed data using 5-part Likert or other quantitative scales from hospice programs across the US. Such data could be used to learn more about the relationship of clinical, functional and nutritional status to life expectancy, thus further refining the methodology of prognosis.

CONCLUSION

Hospice's growth into non-cancer disease is a significant step toward extending end-of-life care to all patients, regardless of diagnosis. Considerable work remains to be done. However, assuming hospice continues to upgrade medical knowledge and skills, and good-faith negotiations continue with Medicare Fiscal Intermediaries to standardize documentation, a workable national system of care for the dying, and its reimbursement, are within our grasp.

NOTES

1. Christakis NA and Escarce JJ. Survival of Medicare patients after enrollment in hospice programs. *N Eng J Med* 1996; 335:172-8.

2. Lynn J, Harrell FE, Cohn F et al. Defining the "terminally ill:" insights from SUPPORT. *Duquesne Law Rev* 1996; 35:311-36.

3. Lynn J, Harrell FE, Cohn F et al. Prognoses of seriously ill hospitalized patients on the days before death: implications for patient care and public policy. *New Horizons* 1997; 5:56-71.

4. Stuart B, Herbst L, Kinsbrunner B et al. *Medical guidelines for determining prognosis in selected non-cancer diseases*, 1st ed. Arlington, VA: National Hospice Organization, 1995.

5. Stuart B, Alexander C, Arenella C et al. *Medical Guidelines for Determining Prognosis in Selected Non-Cancer Diseases*, 2nd ed. *Hospice J* 1995;11:47-63.

6. Thibault GE. Prognosis and clinical predictive models for critically ill patients. In Field MJ and Cassell CK, Eds. *Approaching Death: Improving Care at the End of Life.* Washington DC: National Academy Press, 1997, pp. 358-62.

7. The CONSENSUS Trial Study Group. Effect of enalapril on mortality in severe congestive heart failure: results of the Cooperative North Scandinavian Enalapril Survival Study (CONSENSUS). *N Eng J Med* 1987; 316:1429-35.

8. Unpublished data.

Hospice Care and Palliative Care:
A Perspective from Experience

Paul R. Brenner

SUMMARY. The establishment of the first Department of Pain Medicine and Palliative Care in a Medical Center in the United States is noteworthy. Since the design of the Department integrates a full-functioning hospice program within it, that has both a dedicated inpatient unit and extensive home care program, this Department represents a milestone in the development of the hospice movement, with full interrelationship between palliative care and hospice care. This paper will explore this interrelationship, its implications, and some of the background. *[Article copies available for a fee from The Haworth Document Delivery Service: 1-800-342-9678. E-mail address: getinfo@haworthpressinc. com <Website: http://www.haworthpressinc.com>]*

ORIGINS:
THE HOSPICE MOVEMENT

The origins of the hospice movement in the 1970s in the United States was given impetus in 1974 with the beginning of the first hospice program in New Haven, Connecticut. The organizers of the program incorporated the philosophy and practices carefully developed by Dr. Cicely Saunders and her team at St. Christopher's Hospice, London, and reformed it as essentially a home care service rather than an inpatient care service.

The widespread interest and support hospice received in the 1970s

---

[Haworth co-indexing entry note]: "Hospice Care and Palliative Care: A Perspective from Experience." Brenner, Paul R. Co-published simultaneously in *The Hospice Journal* (The Haworth Press, Inc.) Vol. 14, No. 3/4, 1999, pp. 155-166; and: *The Hospice Heritage: Celebrating Our Future* (ed: Inge B. Corless and Zelda Foster) The Haworth Press, Inc., 1999, pp. 155-166. Single or multiple copies of this article are available for a fee from The Haworth Document Delivery Service [1-800-342-9678, 9:00 a.m. - 5:00 p.m. (EST). E-mail address: getinfo@haworthpressinc.com].

155

was in part due to the work of Elisabeth Kubler-Ross through her books, seminars, and workshops. This was the beginning of a recognition that how dying happened in the United States, especially in medical settings, and needed to change.

The social values of the time were decidedly anti-establishment. There were experimental forms of marriage, family, and community. In religious communities new forms of liturgical expression and music were being created. The women's movement and birthing movements were underway.

The idea of hospice care fell into this fertile environment of ferment for change. The idea of taking dying and death into the family at home and away from the hospital was empowering and liberating. Groups of citizens in communities all across the country took the lead in establishing hospice programs. Although a few farsighted hospitals started hospice programs at this time, they were limited in scope because of the absence of a reimbursement mechanism, as were home health agencies. However, home health agencies in many communities participated in community organizing to start a community-based program. The lack of both reimbursement and dependence upon community resources and volunteers discouraged institutional health care involvement, with a few exceptions.

These early hospice programs usually identified a physician in the community who would serve as medical director, most commonly with very little or no payment for services. Many fine physicians volunteered their time to help these developing community-based hospice programs.

Because the hospice movement largely was a community-based movement, it has had an uneven and undefined relationship with the medical and health care establishments in many communities, even though the community-based hospices worked hard to engage their local medical societies, hospitals, and providers of health care in the care of the dying and their families. Further, the time the community physicians had to give to the hospice program was limited, because most had private practices to manage as well as other responsibilities.

In the United States, therefore, it was often nurses who took leadership roles. Nurses provided not just the primary nursing care, but served as the organizing core of service, providing "case management" which coordinated other services, and were involved as well in providing emotional and spiritual support.

The prototype of this nurse-led model was embodied by the work of Florence Wald, RN, former Dean of the Yale School of Nursing. She organized, advocated, educated, and recruited the group that developed the first American hospice built on the principles Dr. Saunders established at St. Christopher's.

In 1974 with the beginning of the Connecticut Hospice on the East Coast, and in 1976 with the beginning of Hospice of Marin on the West Coast, these two hospices provided learning laboratories through which the philosophy and practice of hospice care spread rapidly in the 1970s and early 1980s, especially as a home care focused program. Basic policies and procedures from these two programs went through many generations of reproduction and expansion. In those years it was common practice for hospices to share information freely, comfortably, and openly with one another.

Central to this early success was the ability of the community-based hospice to attract professional volunteers as well as lay volunteers. In many programs nurses from hospitals volunteered on their off-hours to assist in the care of hospice patients during their off-hours. For example, in Jacksonville, Florida, two nurses would be assigned to one patient to insure there was backup and support, and through volunteer nurses alone, the hospice was able to serve 30 patients in the community. This required a volunteer nursing staff of sixty nurses to maintain.

At that time community-based programs saw their admission criteria as life expectancy measured in months, not years, usually less than a year, but some times more. Patients and families self-selected into hospice, and a strict prognosis was not a requirement in the way it became later under Medicare with its six-month arbitrary point of entry.

With the beginning of State regulation of hospice care, first in Florida, and the addition of hospice as a covered service for Medicare, and then the extension of the benefit to Medicaid in the mid-1980s, more traditional providers of health care began to establish hospice programs. However, the nurse-centered model remained consistent and essential, and was financially viable.

ORIGINS: THE PALLIATIVE CARE MOVEMENT

In her introduction to the *Oxford Textbook of Palliative Medicare* (Saunders, 1993), Dr. Cicely Saunders points to the establishment of hospices (Calvires) in Lyons, France, beginning in 1842. In 1879 in Dublin (Our Lady's Hospice) and in 1905 in London (St. Joseph's Hospice), the Irish Sisters of Charity opened hospices for persons with incurable diseases. Calvary Hospital in New York City began in houses in Greenwich Village in 1899, before moving to the Bronx, using the models in France as inspiration. These hospices provided a "palliative care" approach for persons who were "incurable," often as a "charity."

There were also other similar facilities established by non-Roman Catholic groups at that time. These included the Friedenshein House of Rest, which later was renamed St. Columbus Hospital in 1885, the Hostel of God, which became Trinity Hospice in 1891, and St. Luke's Home for the Dying Poor, which was begun in 1893 to care for persons with tuberculosis as well as cancer.

Dr. Saunders for seven years, beginning in 1948, worked as a volunteer nurse at St. Luke's Home for the Dying Poor, which she acknowledges as a major influence in the planning for St. Christopher's. After completing her medical studies in 1957, she began to work at St. Joseph's Hospital pioneering the use of opioids to control pain and published a series of groundbreaking studies on the results.

In 1967 she opened St. Christopher's Hospice, the first "modern" hospice as we understand the term, with the full support of the National Health Service of Great Britain. As was her practice, Dr. Saunders and her team were engaged in vigorous scientific research from the very beginning to demonstrate the scientific validity of their work.

In the 1970s a unique Palliative Care Program was established at St. Luke's Hospital, New York City (O'Conner, 1998). This program provided a "hospice without walls" within the hospital. A comprehensive Interdisciplinary Team went wherever the patients were, from ER to any nursing unit, to provide full palliative care and end-of-life care. After the decision was made not to apply for certification as a hospice, the program's dependency upon philanthropic support in time made it difficult to support, and it was discontinued by the hospital in the mid-1980s. It was an early creative attempt to put Dr. Saunders principles in place within an American hospital.

Meanwhile, as the hospice movement was emerging and organizing in the late 1970s, at the same time, a group of largely academic-based physicians gathered together to organize the American Pain Society. Dr. John Bonica, Dr. Raymond Houde, and Alice Rogers, RN, were pioneers in the movement, and were to be joined by Kathleen Foley, MD, and Charles Cleeland, PhD, and others.

The Pain Movement became internationally focused, and led to the establishment of the WHO Standards for Cancer Pain Relief, as well as the establishment of State Pain Initiatives in United States (Webb, 1997). Much of this work continues to be physician directed within teaching hospitals, and is based on research.

The Pain Service at Memorial Sloan-Kettering, New York, with Kathleen Foley, M.D., and later Russell Portenoy, M.D., expanded the scope of concern from pain into a broader palliative care perspective. In seeking to manage pain in the course of disease treatment, pain could not often be isolated from other distressing symptoms and problems being experienced by patients. Through the talented team at MSKCC, focused studies were done on other symptoms as well which cause distress.

In 1989, with funding from the Robert Wood Johnson Foundation, the largest study of dying in the United States was begun. The Study to Understand Prognosis and Preferences for Outcomes and Risks of Treatment (commonly called SUPPORT), was a study of 9,000 patients with life threatening medical conditions in five teaching hospitals over a four-year period. The study was to determine the effectiveness of a resource-rich intervention utilizing nurses in an attempt to change how physicians in these five hospitals provided end-of-life care.

After the SUPPORT Study results were published, it is as though the depth and degree of the seriousness of the issues confronting the health care system in providing palliative care at any point in the patient's experience with progressive illness was finally revealed, identified, and acknowledged (Lynn, 1997).

Since SUPPORT, a cluster of activities involving palliative care have been initiated, including:

1. Project On Death In America, The Open Society Institute, The Sorros Foundation.
2. The Hospital Palliative Care Initiative, United Hospital Fund, New York.
3. LAST ACTS Initiative, Robert Wood Johnson Foundation.
4. Center to Improve The Care of the Dying. The George Washington University, Washington, D.C.

5. Retrieving Spiritual Traditions In End of Life Care. The Park Ridge Center, Chicago.
6. Support Care of the Dying. A Coalition of Six Roman Catholic Health Care Organizations.
7. Physician Education Program In End of Life Care, American Medical Association, Chicago.
8. Attorney General's Commission on Quality Care at the End of Life, New York State.
9. Establishment of Department of Pain Medicine and Palliative Care, Beth Israel Medical Center, New York.

NEW CONFIGURATION AT BETH ISRAEL

These two phenomena, Hospice Care and Palliative Care, came together in a new configuration in September, 1997, at Beth Israel Medical Center in New York City.

Jacob Perlow Hospice, established in 1988 by the Beth Israel Medical Center, was the first hospice in New York under the auspices of a Jewish hospital. It was incorporated as a separate entity in order to manage clinical, regulatory and fiscal issues. A group of Trustees from the Medical Center's Board of Trustees was constituted as the Trustees of the Hospice Corporation.

From the beginning it was designed as a comprehensive hospice program, with a dedicated eight-bed inpatient unit, and home care. In its first ten years the hospice functioned much like a community-based hospice rather than an integrated service of the Medical Center. Most of its referrals came from outside its own system, and Beth Israel's main hospital had about twice the number of deaths each year from disease-related causes as did Beth Israel's own hospice.

The Hospice's Medical Director, who had previously been the Medical Director of the Palliative Care Program at St. Luke's Hospital, had not designated or recognized status or role within the Hospital's Department of Medicine. He had unsuccessfully lobbied, year after year, to have the new House Staff have a rotation through the Hospice Unit or to present Grand Rounds on pain control at the end of life.

It seemed reasonably clear that a new configuration was needed. Initial planning started with the Medical Center's Medical Director and the Vice President for Medical Affairs. In 1995 the Hospice's Advisory Board approved a proposal to expand or create through the

Hospice an adjunct palliative care program for in-reach at the Hospital.

The announcement of the United Hospital Fund (UHF) Hospital Palliative Care Initiative came as this work was under way. Beth Israel was awarded a UHF planning grant and later an implementation grant. The project at this time called for the creation of a Palliative Care Interdisciplinary Consultation Team, with prominent medical leadership.

In the course of the search for appropriate physician leadership, Dr. Russell Portenoy became involved in the process. Dr. Portenoy recommended that the Hospital commit to an even bolder plan: create a Department for Pain Medicine and Palliative Care, in doing so, it hired Dr. Portenoy to be the chair.

Jacob Perlow Hospice was at that time administratively moved into the Department to be the end-of-life care provider for the Division of Palliative Care. As a full functioning, financially viable program, the Hospice brought the structures of a donor base, strong outpatient care service, an existing inpatient unit which could be expanded to include palliative care patients, a 24-hour on-call system, which could be extended to other Department home care patients, as well as other systems and experience.

The physicians, advanced practice nurses, and social workers who were brought into the Department brought palliative care and chronic pain management expertise from acute care settings across the country, sophistication and experience in research, and comfort in working within an academic medical model.

However, as was quickly discovered, although similar terminology and concepts existed between the hospice and non-hospice personnel, the words did not always mean the same nor reflect a common "culture" or value "weight" in terms of actual practice.

The nonhospice "culture" is physician-led and physician-directed, while hospice "culture" is nursing-led and nursing-coordinated with leadership more shared within a team which works for consensus. The nonhospice culture has been nurtured in the acute care environment with its focus on aggressive intervention, physician orders, hierarchical structuring of care, and dealing with patients only at a time of acute crisis. Hospice culture has been more reflective, utilizing an active listening approach to clarify underlying patient/family needs and problems as well as what shows, and serves patients as well as families across a much longer diverse period of time.

Non-hospice medical "culture" has dealt most frequently with patients who were still in active disease treatment and whose goals of care and course of therapy reflect life-extension, while the hospice "culture" has only dealt with persons whose basic tasks involve finding an appropriate self-determined closure to life and all the complex issues and problems that surround it.

As these differences surfaced in different arenas and situations, a Change and Transition Committee was formed, with key representatives from the Pain Division, the Palliative Care Division, and the Hospice. This Committee worked through intricate issues of finding unity within these different cultures, in order to build an underlying consensus and commonality, as well as identified structures to assist staff members deal with conflicts and differences. Of great importance to the Committee's work was identifying unifying values.

New to the hospice staff was the vigorous focus on evidence-based care, physician involvement and physician interest in participating actively in managing the details of care. New to many of the nonhospice staff, especially physicians, was the practice of managing care "from a distance." Since over 90% of hospice care is delivered at home, often with patients who are very ill and immobile, Department physicians had to learn how to be comfortable in depending on the skill of nurses to assess problems and communicate them accurately to physicians.

DISTINCT CHALLENGES
TO JACOB PERLOW HOSPICE STAFF

One distinct challenge for Jacob Perlow Hospice at many levels relates to a cluster of issues involved in the loss of autonomy for its existence and control of its own destiny. Now as a part of a larger continuum of care and a Department in the Medical Center, decisions cannot be made as simply and quickly as before, funding opportunities must be negotiated carefully, and, at times, compromised, and systems are more complex.

While the delivery of hospice care is care at the end of life, the Hospice is part of a Department with a much broader scope of care and interest. Hospice personnel on the inpatient unit and providing on-call services needed training and skills building to manage patients with diverse goals of care. The loss of a single focus for all care was particularly challenging for some inpatient nurses.

While palliative care is not regulated, hospice care is presently tightly regulated. To create an integrated model of care while continuing to meet all conditions of participation and regulatory requirements has been particularly challenging. The new "compliance" environment involving the Office of the Inspector General (OIG) and Medical Review Guidelines has added to the complexity.

The hospice management and supervisory staff has had the task of providing direction and support to the hospice clinical staff, whose identity, roles, relationships, and positions are undergoing change and redefinition. It has not only been stressful to the hospice clinical staff but its management staff as well. Some staff members have been more comfortable and adept at discovering opportunities for collaboration and expansion into palliative care than others.

At the clinical level, nurses, social workers, chaplains, other therapists, and volunteer coordinators, who have seen themselves as experts in hospice care, have been required to learn new skills in assessing and managing patients, and integrate "evidence-based" thinking into their practice. For the homecare nursing staff this has strengthened their ability to communicate treatment options more effectively to physicians in the community. It has changed the dynamic of the relationship from being one of what the nurse wants to do versus what evidence says is the best way to proceed. That approach carries more authority with physicians.

CHALLENGES TO DEPARTMENT PALLIATIVE CARE PROFESSIONALS

Distinct challenges to the palliative care physicians, nurses, and social workers in learning how to integrate with hospice involved mastery of the technical requirements for hospice regarding prognosis, how hospice finances work, how the interdisciplinary team functions, and the necessity for ongoing clear communication.

While the goal of palliative care is to provide the diverse, broad array of services hospice provides before the end of life and throughout the process of disease management, it is difficult and challenging to do this within the existing reimbursement structure. It is especially difficult to provide all the psychosocial, spiritual, and existential support that patients and families need along the way prior to end-of-life care, and especially in the outpatient community environment.

Palliative care has developed a research agenda which it knows how to manage in the acute care setting, but has less experience in organizing and managing in outpatient and home care settings. The challenge of how to incorporate hospice issues into a research agenda and funding is critical in an integrated system, such as the Department.

While palliative care has placed great emphasis on evidence-based care, that is, what research determines is best practice for the desired outcomes, it has not focused as much attention as has the hospice on individual "practice models," that is, how the personal and professional interact in one's ongoing clinical engagement with patients and family members. The long rich experience of hospice with staff support is not as much a part of the palliative care experience to date, and the creation of effective adequate support structures which include its physicians is a major challenge to be addressed.

ADVANTAGES OF A PALLIATIVE CARE CONTINUUM TO HOSPICE

As with much of the rest of the hospice community, Jacob Perlow Hospice up until 1997 had experienced an ongoing steady reduction in length of stay, both by average length of stay for all patients and median length of stay. This shortened length of stay has compressed the care of patients and families to a time of profound crisis which requires multiple services to manage the crisis, and prevents the elegance that hospice can bring at life's end from being routinely available. In addition, like other hospices, the integration of decertification into its care management strategy, as fiscal intermediary oversight requires documented evidence of ongoing specific decline, was stressful to staff and disruptive to good patient care. Finally, reduced length of stay and the compression of care has increased the cost of care without an increase in reimbursement to cover that expense.

In addition, New York City is a health care environment of great diversity, complexity, overlapping and at times conflicting systems of care. Hospice care is not the only viable choice in the community for end-of-life care. Calvary Hospital and Rivington House are two examples of institutional alternatives, one for cancer and one for AIDS. In addition, non-hospice home care programs can easily place 24 hour attendant care at home for long periods of times. In AIDS care, the costs of all drugs are "carved out" of the payment structure and can be billed separately. Within this environment hospice care is at a distinct disadvantage, in spite of its experience, expertise and satisfactory outcomes in end of life care.

To the leadership of Jacob Perlow Hospice, these issues were also a significant factor in changing the status of the hospice from an independent "outsider" to an integrated "insider" in its own system. One of the fundamental assumptions that was made in creating the Department was that the pain and palliative care professionals, as a result of consultations, clinics, and office visits, would connect with patients and families the hospice could not connect with, and that would happen earlier in the end-of-life phase of their illness. As the Department grows and the hospital learns how to use the Department, patients will be referred into hospice care, who before, would not have had that referral at all, and the length of time of their experience with hospice care will increase. The overall expectation is that hospice length of stay will increase and patients and families will arrive increasingly having already dealt with transition issues. As a welcomed side benefit, the financial stress of managing hospice will decrease.

After the first year of the Department's existence, when it went from one nonhospice staff member to over twenty, the median length of stay in hospice care reversed for the first time. It increased from a low of 17 days in 1997 to almost 23 days by 1999. This seems to confirm the basic assumption that was made, and that positive change has occurred.

CONCLUSION

As the Department enters its second year of integration, the primary challenges involve how to manage its development, how to expand resources so it has presence throughout the health care system of which it is a part, and how to develop a common culture of shared values and community between the hospice personnel and those who come from nonhospice settings.

At the same time whether the hospice movement at large can successfully address some of its key issues: six month prognosis, medical review guidelines for prognosis and recertification, "benefit creep," (i.e., payor expectation that hospice absorbs costs for services not considered in 1984, example, Protease Inhibitors for AIDS patients), and the rigidity of the four levels of care, will also affect the ability of Jacob Perlow Hospice, as part of a continuum of palliative care, to play an expanded role in patient and family care within the Department, the System's Hospitals, its Ambulatory Care Center, and its System's Home Health Agency.

However, the greatest issue for the Department with Hospice is its charge from the Beth Israel Board of Trustees to be an agent for changing the basic culture of the Medical Center and its Health Care System away from "practice" which is represented by SUPPORT to the more humane, comprehensive, patient-family centered "practice," characterized by hospice and palliative care.

REFERENCES

Information from Interview with Sr. Patrice O'Conner, Director of the Palliative Care Program, St. Luke's Hospital, New York City, 1998.

Lynn, J. "Unexpected Returns: Insights From SUPPORT, " *The Robert Wood Johnson Foundation Anthology.* San Francisco: Jossey-Bass Publishers, 1997.

Saunders, C. *Oxford Textbook On Palliative Medicine.* Oxford: Oxford University, Press, 1993.

Webb, M. *The Good Death: The New American Search to Reshape the End of Life.* New York: Bantam Books, 1997.

Putting Patient and Family Voice Back into Measuring Quality of Care for the Dying

Joan M. Teno

SUMMARY. Quality of care and quality of life change substantially for those with a serious chronic illness and nearing the end of their lives. As one dies, life takes on new shape–values change and things once ignored become more important. Existing quality of care measures do not attend to the changes in priorities or to dimensions that acquire new significance (e.g., Spirituality and transcendence). An important impediment to addressing the inadequacies in the evidence base for palliative care, improving shortcomings of care, and holding institutions or health care systems accountable for the quality of care is the lack of valid and reliable measurement tools. In this article, an overview is presented of an ongoing research effort to develop measurement tools which will utilize the patient and family perspective to measure the quality of care. *[Article copies available for a fee from The Haworth Document Delivery Service: 1-800-342-9678. E-mail address: getinfo@haworthpressinc.com <Website: http://www.haworthpressinc.com>]*

KEYWORDS. Quality of care, measurement, terminal illness

INTRODUCTION

THIS IS MY WORLD NOW. IT'S ALL I HAVE LEFT. YOU SEE. I am old. And, I'm not as healthy as I used to be. I'm not necessarily happy with it, but I accept it.

[Haworth co-indexing entry note]: "Putting Patient and Family Voice Back into Measuring Quality of Care for the Dying." Teno, Joan M. Co-published simultaneously in *The Hospice Journal* (The Haworth Press, Inc.) Vol. 14, No. 3/4, 1999, pp. 167-176; and: *The Hospice Heritage: Celebrating Our Future* (ed: Inge B. Corless and Zelda Foster) The Haworth Press, Inc., 1999, pp. 167-176. Single or multiple copies of this article are available for a fee from The Haworth Document Delivery Service [1-800-342-9678, 9:00 a.m. - 5:00 p.m. (EST). E-mail address: getinfo@haworthpressinc.com].

. . . Why do you think the staff insists on talking baby talk when speaking to me? I understand English. I have a degree in music and am a certified teacher . . . I tried once or twice to make my feelings known. I even shouted once. That gained me a reputation of being "crotchety." Imagine me, crotchety. My children never heard me raise my voice. I surprised myself. After I have asked for help more than dozen times . . . something begins to break. That time I wanted to be taken to a bathroom. . . . Something else that I learned to accept is a loss of privacy. Quite often, I'll close my door when my roommate–imagine having a roommate at my age–is in the TV room . . . As I sit thinking or writing, one of the aides invariably opens the door unannounced and walks in as if I'm not there. Some times she opens my drawers and begins rummaging around. Am I invisible? Have I lost my right to respect and dignity? I am still a human being. I would like to be treated as one.

Anna Mae Halgrim Seaver, who lived in Wauwtosa, Wis., died in March. Her son found these notes in her room after her "death." Published in *Newsweek*, June 27, 1994, page 11.

At the heart and the purpose of medicine is healing and caring for human beings. Unlike a business that manufactures widgets, medicine provides a vital service that has a dramatic impact on the lives of persons and their loved ones. Similar to widget manufacturers, however, we must utilize tools that measure and examine the degree to which medical services produce results that are valued by consumers and society as a whole. We can't throw our hands up in the air and say, "trust me, I produce quality medical care." Rather, we must measure our "end results" and constantly strive to improve them. How do we measure our "end results"? Is it just that the rate of pain is less than a 4 out of 10? Is it how many patients die with decubitus ulcers? What is fundamental to caring for such a vulnerable population is acknowledging the need to listen to both the dying person and their family about both technical and caring aspects of medical care. Even if Mrs. Seaver's nursing home in Wauwtosa had the lowest rate of decubitus ulcers, there is a very important problem with the quality of medical care. Such a problem with the quality of care can only be remedied by listening and responding to the patient's voice.

Donabedian noted that "achieving and producing health and satisfaction, as defined for its individual members by a particular society or subculture, is the ultimate validator of the quality of care" (Donabedian, 1966). The Institute of Medicine defined quality of care as "the degree to which health services for individuals and populations increase the likelihood of desired health outcomes and are consistent with current professional knowledge" (IOM, 1990, p. 21). Central to both of these definitions is a person's voice–their preferences, desires, expectations or satisfaction with medical care services delivered. Satisfaction or more appropriately the measurement of satisfaction has recently fallen in disrepute. We have all been bombarded with billboards that proclaim that 98% of Acme Health Plan members feel "We provide excellent medical services" or the chief operating officer who proudly proclaims to a board of directors that since the merger of Home Health Plan A and Hospice B 89% of our consumers state, "We do an excellent job." Lost in this hyperbole is the response rate of 11% or that the discriminate validity of many used satisfaction measures are suspect. This should not lead us to cast aside the patient voice concerning the quality of medical care. The patient voice is central to the care of dying persons. The ability to listen to older persons, educate them about their illness, learn from them, and help guide them through important life choices that balance quality of life concerns with patient longevity is at the core of both geriatric and palliative care medicine.

In this essay, I will provide a brief overview of current problems with measuring satisfaction, and suggest a taxonomy for classification of measurement tools to incorporate the patient and family perspective about the quality of care. Finally, I will outline a research agenda for developing new measurement tools that focus on the perceptions of quality of care from the perspective of the patient and their loved ones. A central tenet of this paper is that the most important outcome variable for examining the quality of care of the dying is whether health care providers understood and responded to the expectations and preferences of the dying patient and their loved ones (Teno, 1996; Teno, 1997).

WHY ARE WE DISSATISFIED WITH CURRENT SATISFACTION MEASURES?

A typical satisfaction measure asks a person to rate a particular service either on a scale of "excellent to poor" or state how satisfied they were choosing from "very satisfied to very dissatisfied." The person must perform a mental calculation that assesses recall or perceptions about the service provided and their expectations (or preferences) about that service. The use of these satisfaction measurement tools has been problematic for several reasons. Many persons utilize only the two best categories, even when medical care was less than optimal. For example, Williams and Calan found that 95% of persons were satisfied with medical care, yet 38% reported that they had difficulty discussing personal problems with their physician and 35% felt that the physician did not spend enough time with them (Williams and Calan, 1991). Furthermore, the fundamental assumption is that the difference between "very good" and "excellent" is the same as the difference between "fair" and "poor." This assumption may not hold (Fowler, 1996). Getting a very good response may be just the tip of the iceberg, indicating an important opportunity to improve and enhance medical care. A response of "good" may indicate a serious concern.

Another important concern is the degree in which a person feels empowered to or choose to voice concerns about their quality of medical care, even to an anonymous interviewer over the phone (Vouri, 1987). This concern is most likely more significant for persons receiving long term care service, an extremely vulnerable population dependent on providers for basic needs. Another important concern is reduced expectations. In a study of seriously ill and dying patients, Desbiens and colleagues found that the majority of patients stated that they were "very satisfied" despite pain that was extremely or moderately severe for one half or more of the time (Desbiens, 1996). In an audit of patients who died in an inner city managed care organization, we specifically asked surviving loved ones whether they thought anything could have been done to improve pain management. Invariably, family members who reported severe pain would state that *"The doctors did all that they could"* (Teno, under review). Yet, research evidence indicates that between 70 and 90% of patients' pain can be palliated with the option of sedation to provide relief for the remaining persons (Schug, 1990; Zech, 1995; Portenoy, 1994; Truog, 1992). Lowered expectations and the lack of knowledge about or regarding what is possible is an important limitation to the validity of patient response to questionnaires asking them to rank aspects of their medical care. Furthermore, patient reports of technical quality may be overly based on the interpersonal skills of the provider. For example, highly empathic skills may mask poor medical judgments.

These and other important problems have been identified with satisfaction measurements (Ware, 1978; Rubin, 1990; Walker,1984; Ley, 1976; Cleary 1988; Kavitz 1998; Rosenthal, 1997; Ross, 1995; Zinn, 1993; Jackson and Kroenke, 1997; Ware, 1988; Aharony and Strasser, 1993). Indeed, satisfaction measures have been referred to now as a "trivial pursuit." The word "satisfaction" has now been applied to a variety of measurement tools, such that we are now increasingly confused and unable to answer the question, "what is satisfaction?"

NEED OF A NEW TAXONOMY
OF MEASURING THE PATIENTS' VOICE

Dying persons and their loved ones provide a very important perspective in judging the quality of care delivered them. Speaking with patients can only assess several aspects of the quality of care. The unifying goal of these measures is incorporating the dying person and loved ones perspective or voice on the quality of care (see Figure 1). Three main strategies have been used in measuring the consumer voice or perspective of the quality of care. Traditionally, we have relied on patients' ranking or ratings of the quality of care. For the most part, these measures have been criticized because of their skewed distribution, acquiescence response bias, and problems with reduced consumer expectations. Preference based assessment (or indirect assessment of satisfaction) has grown out of a long tradition of examining the quality of care based on a persons reports of unmet needs or desire for additional services (Hughes 1998, Manton 1988, Wolisky and Johnson, 1991). Similar to rankings, reduced patient expectations may limit their validity. Furthermore, preferences may be both ethereal and ephemeral–an important concern being the instability of those wishes. Few studies have examined the stability of patient reports.

Cleary and colleagues responding to concerns about patient rankings of the quality of care created "patient centered reports." Questions were framed, "to be as specific as possible, to minimize the influence of confounding factors such as patient expectations, personal relationship, gratitude, or response tendencies related to gender, class or ethnicity (Cleary, Health Affairs, 1991). As indicated in Figure 1, these reports either ask the patient a factual question (e.g., "If you

FIGURE 1. Proposed Classification Scheme for Measuring a Patient Voice About Their Quality of Medical Care

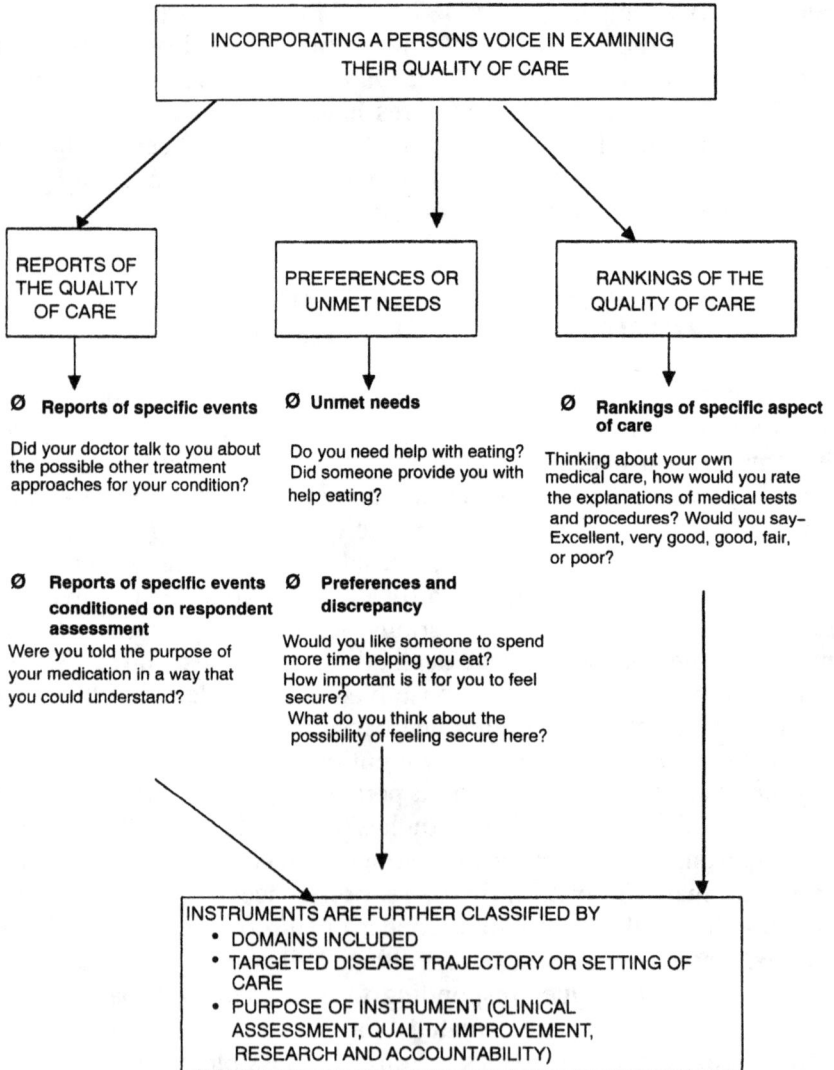

INCORPORATING A PERSONS VOICE IN EXAMINING THEIR QUALITY OF CARE

REPORTS OF THE QUALITY OF CARE

PREFERENCES OR UNMET NEEDS

RANKINGS OF THE QUALITY OF CARE

Ø **Reports of specific events**

Did your doctor talk to you about the possible other treatment approaches for your condition?

Ø **Unmet needs**

Do you need help with eating? Did someone provide you with help eating?

Ø **Rankings of specific aspect of care**

Thinking about your own medical care, how would you rate the explanations of medical tests and procedures? Would you say– Excellent, very good, good, fair, or poor?

Ø **Reports of specific events conditioned on respondent assessment**

Were you told the purpose of your medication in a way that you could understand?

Ø **Preferences and discrepancy**

Would you like someone to spend more time helping you eat? How important is it for you to feel secure? What do you think about the possibility of feeling secure here?

INSTRUMENTS ARE FURTHER CLASSIFIED BY
- DOMAINS INCLUDED
- TARGETED DISEASE TRAJECTORY OR SETTING OF CARE
- PURPOSE OF INSTRUMENT (CLINICAL ASSESSMENT, QUALITY IMPROVEMENT, RESEARCH AND ACCOUNTABILITY)

had to wait to get to your room, did someone from the hospital explain the reason for the delay?") or asks the person to judge one specific aspect of their medical treatment (e.g., "Were you told of the purpose of your medications in a way that you could understand?").

ARE CONSUMER PERCEPTIONS THE MOST IMPORTANT OUTCOME VARIABLE FOR DYING PATIENTS AND THEIR FAMILIES?

For dying persons, the important concern may not be adding quantity but maintaining their quality of life. Mortality rates or weight loss may not reflect what is important to the patient. For the 45 year-old suffering from an acute myocardial infarction, the vast majority of persons will want medical care that focuses on life extension and myocardial preservation. This does not necessarily hold for the 68 year-old with metstatic colon cancer. Patients reasonably differ in their preferred approach to care. Key to dying persons is that medical care is tailored to their needs and expectations. Too often, the reality is that the organizational needs are put first prior to those of the patient and their loved ones. We must demand of our health care system that medical care must be patient focused and family centered. Measurement tools that ascertain the patient and family perspective are an important step in ensuring that medical care focuses not only on the technological aspects of care, but on humanistic or caring aspects. This is our primary goal in the development of new measurement tools for the Toolkit of Instrument to Measure End-of-Life Care (TIME).

PRIORITIES FOR FUTURE DEVELOPMENT OF TOOLKIT OF INSTRUMENTS TO MEASURE END-OF-LIFE CARE (TIME)

A central goal of the Toolkit is that measures incorporate the patient and loved ones perspective, be clinically meaningful, and strive for high standards of reliability, validity, and responsiveness. Our initial focus is on developing tools for ongoing monitoring of quality of care based on both the patient's and loved ones' report on the processes of care that are delivered to them. In developing TIME, we will mainly rely on the methodology of patient centered reports to examine whether key processes were done in a means beneficial to patients and their loved ones. Determining what the key processes are will be informed by existing guidelines (e.g., Canadian Palliative Care Association Towards a Consensus in Standardized Principles of Practice) and focus groups with terminally ill patients and their loved ones. Our aim is that the created instruments will initially be used in conducting audits and improving the quality of care of persons diagnosed with life threatening illness, that is expected to be fatal. Hence, our focus will be on face or content validity of the instrument to measure clinically important aspects of providing medical care for a vulnerable population.

Our vision is that there will be a core instrument with additional modules that will allow potential users to design a tool to fit their own institutional needs. While the domains to be included in the instrument will be informed based on the planned focus groups preliminary data gathered from the review of existing focus groups and discussions with participants at two conferences, provided the insight into the development of the TIME. The following is an initial list based on the review and discussions: (1) communication, decision-making, and advance care planning; (2) symptom management; (3) organizational responsiveness to the patient and their loved ones; (4) bereavement and psychological support; (5) coordination and continuity of medical care; and (6) personal meaning, transcendence, and spirituality. The final "Toolkit" will have measurement tools, suggestions for the preparation of actionable reports, and a resource guide. The resource guide will provide information on the use of the instruments, interpreting results, and taking the next steps to improve the quality of care.

If we are going to improve the quality of care of the dying, what is needed are measurement instruments which assess the quality of care captured from the perspective of the dying persons and their loved ones. Only patients and their loved ones can report on important aspects of the quality of care that was delivered to them. Key is that medical care meets the patients and family needs and that they are treated with dignity and respect. Mrs. Anna Mae Halgrim Seaver posed the question, "Am I invisible? Have I lost my right to respect and dignity?" Our answer must be a resounding no. For Mrs. Seaver, the only persons that can provide such intimate and crucial information are she and her family.

REFERENCES

Aharony L, Strasser S. (1993). Patient Satisfaction: What we know about and what we still need to explore. *Med Care Rev,* 50 (1), 49-79.

Cleary PD, Edgman-Levitan S, Roberts M et al. (1991). Patients evaluate their hospital care: A national survey. *Health Aff, 10,* 254-267.

Cleary PD, McNeil BJ. (1988) Patient satisfaction as an indicator of quality care. *Inquiry,* 25, 25-36.

Desbiens N, Wu AW, Broste SK et al. (1996) Pain and satisfaction with pain control in seriously ill hospitalized adults: findings from the SUPPORT research investigations. For the SUPPORT investigators. Study to Understand Prognoses and Preferences for Outcomes and Risks of Treatment. *Critical Care Medicine, 24,* (12), 1953-61.

Fowler FJ, Jr., Barry MJ, Lu-Yao G, Wasson JH, and Bin L. (1996) Outcomes of External Beam Radiation Terapy for Prostrate Cancer: A Study of Medicare Beneficiaries on Three Seer Areas. *Journal of Clinical Oncology, 14* (8), 2258-65.

Hughes S, Conrad K, Mannheim L et al. (1988) Impact of long-term home care on mortality, functional status, and unmet needs. *Health Serv Res,* 23, 269-294.

Institute of Medicine. (1990). Medicare: A strategy for quality assurance. Washington, DC: National Academy Press.

Jackson, JL, Kroenke K. (1997). Patient satisfaction and quality of care. *Mil Med 162* (4), 273-277.

Kravitz R. (1998). Patient satisfaction with health care: Critical outcome or trivial pursuit? *J Gen Intern Med,* 13, 280-282.

Ley P, Kinsely J and Atherton ST. (1976). Increasing Patients' Satisfaction with Communication. *British Journal of Social and Clinical Psychology,* 15, 403-413.

Manton KG. (1998). A longitudinal study of sectional change and mortality in the United States. *J Gerontol: Soc Sci,* 43, S153-S161.

Portenoy RK, Thaler HT, Kornblith AB et al. (1994). Symptom prevalence, characteristics and distress in a cancer population. *Qual Life Res,* 3, 183-89.

Rosenthal GE, Shannon SE. The use of patient perceptions in the evaluation of health-care delivery systems. *Med Care,* 35(11), NS58-NS68.

Ross CK, Steward CA, Sinacore JM. (1995). A comparative study of seven measures of patient satisfaction. *Med Care,* 33 (4), 392-406.

Rubin HR. (1990). Can patients evaluate the quality of hospital care? *Med Care Rev* 47(3), 267-326.

Schug SA, Zech D, Dorr U. (1990). Cancer pain management according to the WHO Analgesic Guidelines. *J Pain Symptom Managed,* 5, 27-32.

Teno JM, Landrum KM, Kreling BA, Boekoloo B. (1988). Breaking through the glass ceiling: Is it enough? (manuscript under review).

Teno JM, Landrum K, Lynn J. (1997). Defining and measuring outcomes in end-stage dementia. *Alzheimer Disease and Associated Disorders,* 11, Suppl. 6, 25-29.

Teno, JM. (1996). Consumer reports and ratings of medical care: Will we ever get satisfaction? Institute of Medicine Conference: Evaluating Health Outcomes for Elderly People in a Changing Health Care Marketplace, Briefing Book.

Teno JM, Byock I, Field MA. Research Agenda for Developing Measures to Examine Quality of Care and Quality of Life of Patients Diagnosed with Life Limiting Illness (In Press, *Journal of Pain and Symptom Management*).

Truog RD, Berde CB, Mitchell C, Grier HE. (1992). Barbiturates in the care of the terminally ill. *New England Journal of Medicine*, 327, 1678-1682.

Vouri H. (1987). Patient Satisfaction–An Attribute or Indicator of the Quality of Care? Editorial. *Quality Review Bulletin*, 13, 106-8.

Walker AH, Restuccia JD. (1984). Obtaining Information on Patient Satisfaction with Hospital Care: Mail versus Telephone. *Health Services Research*, 19, 291-396.

Ware JE. (1978). Effects of acquiescent response set on patient satisfaction ratings. *Med Care*, (4), 327-336.

Williams SJ, Calnan M. (1991). Convergence and Divergence: Assessing criteria of consumer satisfaction across general practice, dental, and hospital settings. *Soc Sci Med*, 33, 707-716.

Wolinsky F, Johnson R. (1991). The use of health services by older adults. *J Gerontol: Soc Sci*, 46, S345-S357.

Zech DF et al. (1995). Validation of World Health Organization guidelines for cancer pain relief: a 10-year prospective study. *Pain*, 63, 65-67.

Documenting the Impact of Hospice

Melanie P. Merriman

SUMMARY. Hospice care has had an impact at many levels–on individual patients and families, on the health care industry, and on society. However, no comprehensive body of evidence has been generated that documents the impact of hospice care in terms that are meaningful to competitors, referral sources, and consumers. In part, this is because of the many challenges for evaluating hospice care. This paper describes recent efforts in the documentation of the value of hospice which have focused on outcomes measurement by individual providers rather than on large scale studies. Several groups are working to develop reliable measurement tools, to support standardized measurement in large numbers of hospices, and to collect information for benchmarking and comparison. Measurement of the impact of hospice care will set standards for other providers of end-of-life care and will document the expertise and knowledge of hospice professionals. Once established as centers of excellence in care of the dying, hospices will be well positioned for whatever delivery models may evolve for end-of-life care. *[Article copies available for a fee from The Haworth Document Delivery Service: 1-800-342-9678. E-mail address: getinfo@haworthpressinc.com <Website: http://www.haworthpressinc.com>]*

KEYWORDS. Hospice, end-of-life care, outcomes measurement, program evaluation

INTRODUCTION

Birthdays, anniversaries, new year celebrations, and end-of-life are times we typically contemplate meaning and impact. Has this year, has

---

[Haworth co-indexing entry note]: "Documenting the Impact of Hospice." Merriman, Melanie P. Co-published simultaneously in *The Hospice Journal* (The Haworth Press, Inc.) Vol. 14, No. 3/4, 1999, pp. 177-192; and: *The Hospice Heritage: Celebrating Our Future* (ed: Inge B. Corless and Zelda Foster) The Haworth Press, Inc., 1999, pp. 177-192. Single or multiple copies of this article are available for a fee from The Haworth Document Delivery Service [1-800-342-9678, 9:00 a.m. - 5:00 p.m. (EST). E-mail address: getinfo@haworthpressinc.com].

my life, meant anything? Was there any impact? For the institution of hospice, on this 20th anniversary of The National Hospice Organization, the answer is a resounding "YES," and yet it seems clear that there is more to do with respect to documenting that impact. The more that regulators, media, and other health care providers focus on care of the terminally ill, the more hospices are challenged to showcase their expertise, even to prove their success in providing high quality, efficient end-of-life care that meets the unique needs of patients and their families.

The following discussion will focus on four questions: What does it mean to demonstrate the impact of hospice? How has an impact been demonstrated and where are the gaps? What are the challenges and opportunities for moving forward? What current efforts hold the most promise for documenting hospice success and value into the next millennium?

WHAT DOES IT MEAN TO DEMONSTRATE THE IMPACT OF HOSPICE?

The impact of hospice care potentially can be evaluated at several different levels, and would be demonstrated in different ways at each level. In day to day practice at the individual hospice level, the important impact of hospice care is in meeting the needs of terminally ill patients and their families by improving clinical status and maintaining or improving quality of life. At this level, the impact of hospices services can be documented through measurement of clinical, psychosocial, needs fulfillment, and quality of life outcomes. Outcomes measurement is still a relatively new concept in hospice care, but many hospices are now adding this technique to their quality and performance improvement efforts. In a larger context, at the level of the health care industry, the impact of hospice care can be evidenced by alterations in institutions, changes in the knowledge and attitudes of non-hospice health care professionals, and the standardization and professionalization of hospice practice. At a societal level, the impact of hospice care might be seen in changing attitudes about death and dying, a lessening of the fear of the dying process, and greater confidence in the health care system to care compassionately for the dying. Finally, with respect to public policy and the national health care budget, there always has been an expectation that hospice care would have an impact on the costs of care for the dying.

WHAT DEMONSTRATION DO WE HAVE OF THE IMPACT OF HOSPICE AND WHERE ARE THE GAPS?

Hospice is having an impact at all these levels, although documentation of the impact varies. Care of the terminally ill is getting media attention; research in palliative care is attracting new and increased funding; certification is available for nurse and physician palliative care professionals; and hospice care is under scrutiny by federal investigators.

While the latter is disturbing, the reason for federal scrutiny (the growth in the number of patients served from 158,000 in 1985 to a projected 495,000 in 1997) is a powerful demonstration of the impact of hospice. Hospice is one of the fastest growing of Medicare services (33% increase in expenditures between 1990 and 1996),[1] not, I would argue, because of systematic fraud or abuse as has been alleged by the OIG, but because more patients and physicians are aware of the hospice alternative and desire it. On the other hand, patients still come to hospice too late and the length of stay is too short (Christakis and Escarce, 1996). These data suggest that gaps remain in the knowledge of when, in the course of an illness, hospice is an appropriate choice and what hospice expertise can accomplish when there is sufficient time before death. In one effort to close that gap, and to impact care of the terminally ill into the future, hospices are directing or participating in training programs for student nurses and physicians (see, for example, Weissman and Griffie, 1998).

At the individual patient level, the National Hospice Organization (NHO) has conducted a small scale study of pain management and found that on average hospice patients are comfortable with average patient-reported pain severity of 1.89 on a scale of 0 to 10. In addition, the NHO Family Satisfaction Survey, now in use in nearly 350 hospices nationwide, consistently documents high satisfaction with hospice care and services. These data remain, however, preliminary and unpublished, and are not therefore, compelling outside of the industry.

At the societal level, a study by Lewin VHI, Inc., prepared for the National Hospice Organization in 1995, did document a positive impact on cost savings. The study revealed that hospice care costs less than Medicare fee-for-service non-hospice care for similar patients. The study, however, does not address cost comparisons for patients in Medicare HMOs and has been criticized for using the most costly health care (Medicare fee-for-service) as a baseline. Because costs are relatively easy to quantify, this is often one of the first measures of impact applied to a health care delivery model. There is a danger that when cost is the focus, dollars will dominate decision-making, particularly when the issue becomes competition and choices between alternative providers (Iezzoni, 1997). Iezzoni (1997) rightfully appeals for investment in gathering quality information, which is needed to balance the competition equation.

Competition is, in fact, a driving force behind current efforts to collect information that documents the impact and value of hospice care. If hospice care evolved in response to perceived flaws in the "mainstream" medical system, it now appears that efforts to improve terminal care in both acute care and community settings are evolving in part as a backlash to perceived deficiencies in hospice. The SUPPORT study (The SUPPORT Principal Investigators, 1995), which documented serious deficiencies in care of the terminally ill in some of the country's leading academic medical centers, could have generated a rush to hospice, but it didn't. Instead, numerous efforts to remake end-of-life care sprang up. While hospice leaders and experts often participate in these efforts, they are rarely in the position of driving them.

In response to the SUPPORT Study, which was front page news in many major cities, prominent health care advocacy groups, oversight agencies, grantmakers, and professional associations launched efforts to investigate what was wrong with care of the dying and began efforts to improve end-of-life care. Both the American Medical Association[2] and the American Geriatric Society (J. Amer. Ger. Soc., 1997, V.45, 526-527) published lists of the essential elements of quality care at the end of life. Most hospices felt that addressing these elements was exactly what they had been doing for 20 years. What has struck most hospice leaders is the fact that these reforming efforts have NOT turned to hospice more often for knowledge and expertise. In fact, when hospice is mentioned, it is often in the context of its having done a great job (and having some lessons to teach) and yet NOT being the right model for comprehensive EOL care. Reformers of EOL care point out that hospice is too restrictive because of regulations that require a six-month prognosis (difficult to predict with accuracy), regulatory and philosophical policies that force patients to forgo any but palliative treatment (a false choice for patients with reversible, intermittent crises), and a lack of expertise in the care of diseases other than cancer (Lynn, 1997).

Hospice leaders themselves recognize some of these limitations, but they would suggest that one remedy is to expand access to hospice care through regulatory revision, that is, to build on a successful model rather than creating a new one from scratch. The latter is, in fact, what is proposed in many of the reformation circles, and it remains to be seen how well hospice, as we know it in 1999, will survive.

The question, then, is why didn't "the reformers" immediately turn to hospice for direction in improving end-of-life care? One answer is that while there are several published studies demonstrating a positive impact of hospice care in improving physical status, emotional status, grief resolution, and family satisfaction (see Dawson, 1991 for reference to several studies), there is no comprehensive body of evidence based on measures that are meaningful and valuable both in and out of the industry–to consumers, referral sources, potential competitors. For example, imagine the SUPPORT study (SUPPORT Principal Investigators, 1995) had been conducted in six prominent hospices (rather than hospitals)–what would the data show with respect to these four measures based on those used in SUPPORT:

1. Patients for whom a preference regarding cardiopulmonary resuscitation (CPR) was known and recorded;
2. Patients with "Do Not Resuscitate" orders more than 2 days prior to death;
3. Patients who spent time (the SUPPORT measure was 10 days) in an intensive care unit;
4. Patients for whom family members reported that the patient was in moderate or severe pain at least 50% of the time.

The emergence of the "new" end-of-life movement has spurred the desire among hospice leaders to share their knowledge and experience and to demonstrate the impact that over 20 years of hospice care has made on dying in America. This may in fact be a golden opportunity to begin efforts that will increase the impact of hospice care even while implementing mechanisms for documenting it.

WHÀT ARE THE CHALLENGES AND OPPORTUNITIES IN DOCUMENTING THE IMPACT OF HOSPICE CARE?

Any current deficiencies in the body of knowledge of the impact of hospice on patients and families, health care, and society are not for lack of trying. The fact is that measuring what happens to patients and families during hospice care is hard to do, and measuring lasting effects of hospice care on the health care industry and society are even harder. Current efforts have in fact spent considerable time defining the unique challenges of this work.

One important and nearly intractable challenge arises from the origins of hospice care. In part, the care system was devised to address elements of the dying experience that are almost inherently not quantifiable. In addition, the goals of care are to meet highly individualized needs, goals and expectations. In this context, it becomes very difficult to define quantifiable measures of impact, particularly at the level of patients and families. Moreover, there are those who feel that the very act of quantification diminishes the hospice model of care, bringing it perilously close to the lab value oriented medicine it was designed to repudiate. As Beresford (1996) pointed out, the challenge is to objectively measure a care experience that is inherently subjective.

Another challenge is the limited number of well-crafted measures. It is difficult to construct instruments that balance clinical relevance and research rigor. Tools that are appealing to clinicians, because they capture the essence of hospice care and provide useful data for care planning, may not meet the researchers' rigorous tests for reliability and validity needed in population studies.

One way to meet these challenges, in the context of documenting impact for external audiences, may be to focus less on measuring the most unique aspects of hospice. It may be more useful to use universally accepted measures of aspects of "dying well" that are based in ethical principles or on consumer research (American Health Decisions, 1997; N. Naierman, American Hospice Foundation, internal document and personal communication). It is generally accepted that, with a few exceptions (so few that they would not skew the data in populations), individuals should not die in pain, alone, or while enduring medical treatments they do not want. Measurements for these aspects of dying may be fairly easily devised, although other challenges remain in their implementation.

In hospice, a major challenge is the population for whom we want to measure the impact of care. Both patients and families are vulnerable and, particularly in the case of patients, only a small percentage can provide self-reported data. In patient-reported measures, then, the data primarily will come from the least disabled subset of patients, a clear violation of sampling methodology. One alternative is to use surrogate reporting, which raises the issue of identification of the most appropriate surrogate. While surrogate reporting may be acceptable to researchers, clinicians often feel that asking either patients or families to provide data for measuring the impact of care is intrusive, given the nature of their current experience. One would hope, however, that measures of pain relief, abandonment, and honoring of treatment preferences (see above) would be part of routine care, even if not used for measuring impact.

Another issue with the patient population is that in their choice of hospice care they are already a non-random sample of the dying. Hence, researchers argue, data demonstrating a certain impact within this population does not necessarily predict that hospice care would have the same impact on patients currently in other care settings. A related issue is risk-adjustment. Because hospices are typically the last care setting encountered, patients bring a lifetime of experience to hospice care. Measures of impact may need to be adjusted for patient characteristics that are outside the control of the hospice, including length of stay, stage of disease, and environmental factors, among others.

Another challenge is that measurement of impact costs money and requires time (more money). Decisions about what to measure and implementation of data collection require special expertise, which hospices may need to obtain. Even smaller hospices will find that they need to invest in computers and software; larger programs may decide to computerize other aspects of clinical care and business operations as well. Several health care software firms are now offering hospice-specific modules. Other costs may be externally driven. As an example, the Joint Commission for Accreditation of Healthcare Organizations (JCAHO) now requires accredited hospices to contract with a data collection and analysis vendor (called a Performance Measurement System) to submit measurement information to the JCAHO.

Despite these challenges, the good news is that the hospice model also offers some advantages for measuring the impact of care for the terminally ill. First, there is no problem identifying the population to be studied. Patients in hospice are, by definition, in a terminal phase and expected to live for six months or less. In other settings, it is very difficult to identify the patients for whom end-of-life care measures should be applied. In addition, hospices are unique in their access to survivors since the family (and close friends) of the patient are part of the unit of care. These individuals are not only accessible, but typically also have first-hand knowledge of the patient's care.

Furthermore, investment in documenting the impact of hospice care offers valuable opportunities for hospice. Through measurement of the effects of hospice, benchmarks will be set for end-of-life care in all settings. For example, in documenting that hospice patients report pain severity of less than 2 (on a scale of 0-10, where 0 = no pain and 10 = worst pain imaginable) in the last month of care (NHO Pain Study, unpublished, 1996), hospice sets a standard that other providers must meet. As described below, several groups, including NHO, are now building on this initial data. Measurement and documentation of other results of hospice care can leverage years of experience and establish hospices as the experts in end-of-life care. The hospice industry undoubtedly will be affected by ongoing changes in health care financing and delivery, and once established as centers of excellence, hospices will be well-placed to participate in, even lead, whatever new models of end-of-life care evolve.

What will it mean to successfully document the impact of hospice care? What will success look like? First, the industry will be able to describe the experience of dying with hospice care for a large patient population, in terms that are meaningful to competitors, referral sources, and consumers. Success would mean that these same groups would point to hospice to illustrate "how people die well." The report of the Institute of Medicine study of end-of-life care (1997) stated that dying patients deserve " . . . skillful compassionate care that reflects their own wishes and those of families. . . ." If the industry believes that this statement describes current hospice care, then success would mean documenting the experience in a way that is irrefutable.

CURRENT EFFORTS

Since the early days of hospice in the U.S., there has been a recognition of the need to document the impact of hospice care (Parks, 1979;

Parks, 1980; Mount and Scott, 1983). The most comprehensive evaluation to date was the National Hospice Study (NHS) of 1981-82, commissioned by HCFA to measure the impact of the Medicare hospice demonstration projects. The results did document a limited impact (National Hospice Study, 1986), and the study was hampered by the lack of instruments designed for use with populations at the end-of-life (Mount and Scott,1983). Beginning in the 1980s, there have been a number of small-scale studies of hospice care, some of which have included the development and/or testing of more suitable evaluation tools. Several studies have also looked at the costs of hospice care (see Scitovsky, 1994), thereby evaluating one aspect of societal impact.

More recent efforts have been shaped by the growing emphasis in health care on outcomes management and performance measurement. Efforts are directed more toward developing evaluation mechanisms that can be implemented by individual hospices, rather than conducting large scale studies to evaluate hospice care from the outside. Hospice professionals and research professionals (from the biomedical, public health, health services and consumer arena) are working separately and sometimes collaborating on projects with three primary objectives: (1) development and implementation of meaningful, valid measures and instruments; (2) standardization of measurement across hospices and other end-of-life care settings; and (3) centralized sharing of outcomes and evaluation data for benchmarking and comparison. One thought is that through collating standardized evaluation data from numerous hospices the information for demonstrating industrywide impact may emerge. It is important to note however that the measures and methodological requirements for internal quality improvement versus external accountability may differ considerably (Solberg et al., 1997).

With respect to instrument and measure development, there has been considerable progress. Hearn and Higginson (1997) reviewed a variety of relatively new instruments for measuring outcomes of palliative care, some of which were developed with hospice patients. At least three quality of life measures specifically designed for patients with terminal illness have been developed in the last 6 years–the Hospice Quality of Life measure (MacMillan and Mahon, 1994), the McGill Quality of Life Index (Cohen and Mount, 1992; Cohen et al., 1995; Cohen et al., 1996), and the Missoula-VITAS Quality of Life Index (Byock and Merriman, 1998). Both the McGill and the Missoula-VITAS tools are being used in practice with hospice patients. In the physical/functional arena, hospice professionals have considered adapting the OASIS (Outcomes and Assessment Information Set) designed for home health patients, for use as an assessment and outcome measure with hospice patients. It now appears, however, that the tool's format and content have limited applicability for hospice patients. Other instruments, such as the Edmonton Symptom Assessment Scale (ESAS) (Bruera et al., 1991), and the Support Team Assessment System (STAS) (Higginson and McCarthy, 1993) seem to hold more promise. Patient and family satisfaction, perhaps the most important outcome measure for end-of-life care, have been the focus of several efforts at the NHO. The NHO Family Satisfaction Survey, developed in 1995, measures several essential facets of hospice care and is now in use at nearly 350 hospices. The NHO research committee is re-evaluating the existing data for possible publication. The committee is also considering revision of the tool and is preparing an instrument to measure patient satisfaction during the course of care.

Within the last two years, several collaborative groups have been formed for the express purpose of developing measures specific either to hospice care or to end-of-life care regardless of setting. The National Hospice Work Group (NHWG) and the NHO, who have collaboratively convened several task forces to address hospice issues in recent years, have charged a task force with development of hospice outcome measures for implementation in hospices nationwide. The Task Force is an outgrowth of the NHO-sponsored group that developed the Pathway for Patients and Families Facing a Terminal Illness, and is developing measures that will reflect the four end-result outcomes of care identified in the pathway. These are (1) safe dying, (2) comfortable dying, (3) self-determined life closure, and (4) effective grieving. The NHWG/NHO task force is defining indicators that best reflect these outcomes and that can be measured simply and accurately in the real world of hospice care. In addition to representation from approximately 15 hospices, the task force includes individuals from JCAHO and HCFA, two agencies who are bringing external pressure on the hospice industry to measure the impact of care as a regulatory and accreditation issue. As members of the task force, these external monitors provide input to assure that new measures have a chance of meeting these agencies' requirements.

Drawing on both the academic literature and the practical experience of task force members, the group has developed four measures, one for each end-result outcome. Two are patient-reported and two are family-reported, following the death. Importantly, the group has also devised implementation protocols with the goal of making measurement manageable in virtually any hospice setting. The measures and protocols are being pilot tested in late 1998 and 1999 and following testing and revision will be released for public use.

Another collaborative effort is addressing one of the most unique facets of hospice care, and one that receives too little attention–bereavement care. In 1996, Connor and McMaster documented the impact of hospice-based bereavement care on the health care use of surviving spouses in an HMO. Duplication of this study outside of managed care is problematic since hospices do not have access to the medical records of patients' spouses. In order to facilitate evaluation of the impact of bereavement care, the Colorado Hospice Organization convened a task force in 1997 to develop an instrument that will assess the need for and the effects of bereavement interventions for surviving primary caregivers. The instrument is based on Worden's four tasks of mourning (Worden, 1991) and is being administered at 3 months and 13 months post death in pilot testing.

A group convened by the American Hospice Foundation is working on a "report card" aimed at hospice consumers, both individuals and group purchasers. This group, called the Hospice Consortium for Quality Care, includes researchers and managers representing 25 hospices of various sizes, that cover 16 states and most regions of the US. The consortium is focused on developing consumer-oriented performance indicators for hospice care, perhaps taking more of a societal view than some of the other groups. The consortium also intends, however, to develop measures that will assist hospices in monitoring quality of care and to define a minimum data set that could be used to assess performance of any end-of-life care provider.

Two other groups are working on comprehensive instruments to evaluate end-of-life care, regardless of provider, and hospice professionals are contributing to the development and testing of these measures. An effort focused on collecting information for consumers (both health care recipients and health care payors) is being conduced by the Foundation for Accountability (FACCT). The goal of their efforts, which are in the beginning stages, is to encourage use of measures that will eventually help consumers make more informed choices.

In an effort focused more on internal quality improvement and clinical evaluation, Joan Teno and colleagues have convened a group of researchers and providers to construct the Toolkit of Instruments to Measure End-of-Life Care (TIME). Conference participants bring expertise in hospice care, palliative medicine, health services research, and consumer needs and values. The TIME project aims to provide a group of instruments (the first generation of which are available on the Internet at *chcr.Brown.edu/pcoc/toolkit.htm*) that will measure quality of care at the end of life, that is "quality of dying." The project also plans to establish a cooperative that will support measurement in individual provider sites and sharing of data. The TIME participants have carefully considered most of the challenges outlined above and are attempting to develop measures that are manageable (can be implemented in current circumstances) and will be valid.

Because both TIME and FACCT are focussed on multiple provider settings, not just on hospices, the resulting tools are not likely to emphasize hospice-specific values or philosophy. As long as they emphasize issues unique to end-of-life, however, the tools may be useful to hospices and may even serve to identify areas where hospice care differs from other providers.

What is particularly encouraging about these instrument development efforts is the informal collaboration between all of the groups mentioned. Several individuals are working on more than one of these task forces and the leaders of the groups are sharing findings. This extraordinary collegiality benefits the process since expertise and discoveries are being shared, not needlessly duplicated. In the end, the tools developed by all these efforts are therefore very likely to be compatible, if not synergistic.

All of the instrument development efforts also have the objective of widespread implementation, standardization of measurement, and data sharing through a third party for benchmarking and comparison purposes. Two groups, the NHO and the Ohio Hospice Organization (OHO), have already implemented data collection and feedback on a wide scale including tens to hundreds of hospices.

The OHO data project includes nearly 50 hospices of all sizes who serve patients in Ohio. Hospice caregivers collect data from patients about pain severity and quality of life, using standardized and validated instruments. All hospices follow the same protocol for data collection and record the information on scannable forms that are submitted to a third party research company that provides data entry, analysis and feedback services. Recently, the Ohio hospices received collated data for the first year of the project. All participants received graphic and tabular reports showing the outcomes for all the hospices as a group and for their individual hospice. The data revealed that, on average, patients admitted with pain are finding relief and reporting pain at an acceptable level within 48 hours of admission, and patients experience increased quality of life over the course of their care. Individual hospices are benchmarking their data against the group results and using the information for internal quality improvement. The OHO is using the data to document the impact of hospice care within the state and to support increased marketing efforts. The group is now looking at adopting the measures to meet the requirements for JCAHO ORYX reporting.

WHAT NOW, WHAT NEXT?

Documenting the impact of hospice care will require investment in the measurement process at national, local, and individual program levels. Hospice programs must allocate funds for information technology (some kind of computerized data storage and analysis), staff training, and expertise (possibly requiring a new FTE). The benefits of this investment will be immediate, in the form of better information for patient care and quality improvement, and will continue for years in the form of great marketing information. At the local and national levels, hospice associations, organizations and alliances will need to invest in third party data collection for benchmarking and in providing education and support for member hospices.

As individual hospices get better at documenting the impact of hospice at the level of patient and family, national efforts can shift to larger studies designed to measure impact at the health care industry and societal and public policy levels. For example, it may be possible to identify and compare communities that have higher versus lower usage of hospice care. How do they differ demographically and with respect to health care delivery? Are there differences in the physician attitudes, knowledge and behaviors regarding death and dying? Are there differences in community attitudes about death and dying? Do they differ in their understanding and acceptance of hospice care? Do the differences reflect the impact of hospice care, and/or do they indicate ways that hospice can integrate better into a community? Work of Wennberg and colleagues (1998) suggests that the number of hospital beds within a community is a determining factor in whether people die at home or in the hospital. A community study might reveal whether hospice is also a determining factor.

The Missoula Demonstration Project (MDP) is a unique study that provides an instructive model for societal level evaluation. The project seeks to change the experience of death and dying in Missoula, Montana and will involve many elements of the community–hospitals, churches, schools, artists, and others. They have adopted and developed instruments for evaluating community knowledge, attitudes and behaviors at a baseline and will apply them again in 5 and 10 years to observe the impact of the MDP interventions. While we have no real baseline for measuring the impact of hospice care, these kinds of tools could be applied in the kind of community comparison described above.

As previously mentioned, it may also be useful to conduct a mirror version of the SUPPORT Study in a sample of hospice programs. In a year 2000 version of the National Hospice Study, a combination of retrospective chart review and prospective survey of hospice patients and their families would document the current experience of dying in hospice. This experience could then be compared with the experience of dying revealed in the SUPPORT Study in order to see the impact of hospice care.

Studies of this magnitude are enormous undertakings that require experienced researchers and high levels of grant funding. The NHO has made outcomes research a top priority and is likely to lead efforts to generate this funding. If studies are designed with input from those who can articulate policy concerns, the resulting data also may be compelling to those who can make regulatory or reimbursement change.

CONCLUSION

Those who work in hospice have ample evidence of its impact in the smiles, hugs, expressions of relief and gratitude, and size of donations from families touched by hospice care. But as hospice becomes more integrated into mainstream medicine, the need arises to prove the value of this form of care to those outside of the industry. Hospice stories, while powerful, cannot reach far enough. Outcomes measurement and quality report cards are the tickets to play in today's health care arena. A choice not to invest in documenting the impact of hospice is a choice to be marginalized within the health care industry.

In 1990, Mor and Masterson-Allen stated "Pioneers of the hospice movement appear to have realized their goal of altering the pattern of care for the terminal cancer patient, in the traditional medical world . . . " Recent events would suggest that the goal remains elusive, especially for non-cancer patients. Documenting the impact of hospice care will bring hospice closer to the goal. To quote songwriter Paul Simon (1990), "Faith is an island in the setting sun. Proof is the bottom line for everyone."

NOTES

1. Health Care Financing Administration, *A Profile of Medicare Chart Book* (1998), p. 34.
2. Elements of Quality Care for Patients in the Last Phase of Life. The Ethics Standards Division, AMA.

REFERENCES

American Health Decisions (1997). *"The Quest to Die with Dignity,"* Appleton, WI: American Health Decisions.

Beresford, L. (1996). Outcomes for hospice. *Hospice Managers Monograph.* Nashville, TN: THA (An association of hospitals and health systems).

Bruera, E., Kuehn, N., Miller, M.J., Selmser, P., and Macmillan, K. (1991). The Edmonton Symptom Assessment System (ESAS): a simple method for the assessment of palliative care patients. *J. Pall Care,* 7(2), 6-9.

Christakis, N.A., and Escarce, J.J. (1996). Survival of Medicare patients after enrolment in hospice. *New Engl. J. Med.,* 335(3), 172-178.

Cohen, S.R., and Mount, B. (1992). Quality of life in terminal illness: Defining and measuring subjective well-being in the dying. *J. Pall. Care,* 8(3), 40-45.

Cohen, S.R., Mount, B., Strobel, M.G., Bui, F. (1995). The McGill quality of life questionnaire: a measure of quality of life appropriate for people with advanced disease. *Palliative Med.,* 9, 207-219.

Cohen, S.R., Mount, B.M., Thomas, J.J.N., Mount, L.F. (1996). Existential well-being is an important determinant of quality of life. *Cancer,* 77(3), 576-586.

Connor, S.R., and McMaster, J.K. (1996). Hospice, bereavement intervention and use of health care services by surviving spouses. *HMO Practice,* 10(1), 20-28.

Dawson, N.J. (1991). Need satisfaction in terminal care settings. *Soc. Sci. Med.,* 32(1), 83-87

Field, M.J. and Cassel, C.K. (ed.) (1997). *Approaching Death: Improving care at the end of life.* Washington, D.C.: National Academy Press.

Hearn, J., and Higginson, I.J. (1997). Outcome measures in palliative care for advanced cancer patients: a review. *J. Pub. Health Med.*, 19(2), 193-199.

Higginson, I.J., and McCarthy, M. (1993) Validity of the support team assessment schedule: do staffs' ratings reflect those made by patients or their families? *Pall. Med.*, 7, 219-228.

Iezzoni, L. (1997). How much are we willing to pay for information about quality of care? *Ann. of Int. Med.*, 126(5), 391-393.

Lynn, J. (1997). An 88-year-old woman facing the end of life. *J. Amer. Med. Assoc.*, 227(20), 1633-1637.

McMillan, S.C., and Mahon, M. (1994). Measuring quality of life in hospice patients using a newly developed Hospice Quality of Life Index. *Quality of Life Res.*, 3, 437-447.

Mor, V., Greer, D.S., and Kastenbaum, R. (1988). *The Hospice Experience.* Baltimore: The Johns Hopkins University Press.

Mor, V., and Masterson-Allen, S. (1990) Comparison of hospice versus conventional care. *Oncology*, 4(7), 85-91.

Mount, B.M. and Scott, J.F. (1983). Whither hospice evaluation. *J. Chronic Dis.*, 36(11), 731-736.

Naierman, N. and Kreling, B. (1997). Towards a Hospice Consumer Report Card. Unpublished. Source: American Hospice Foundation.

National Hospice Study. (1986). *J. Chronic Dis.*, 39(1), 1-62.

Parks, P. (1979). Evaluation of hospice is needed. *Hospitals*, 53(22), 68-70.

Parks, P. (1980). Evaluation of hospice is still needed. *Hospitals*, 54(22), 56.

Scitovsky, A. (1994). The high cost of dying revisited. *Millbank Memorial Find Quarterly*, 72, 561-591.

Solberg, L.I., Mosser, G., and McDonald, S. (1997). The three faces of performance measurement: improvement, accountability and research. *J. Qual. Imp.*, 23(3), 135-147.

The SUPPORT Principal Investigators. (1995). A controlled trial to improve care for seriously ill hospitalized patients: The study to understand prognoses and preferences for outcomes and risks of treatments (SUPPORT). *J. Amer. Med. Assoc.*, 274(20), 1591-1598

Weissman, D.E. and Griffie, J. (1998). Integration of palliative medicine at the Medical College of Wisconsin 1990-1996. *J. Pain and Symp. Mgmt.*, 15(3), 195-201.

Wennberg, J.E. (1998). *The Dartmouth Atlas of Healthcare.* Chicago: Amer. Hops. Publishing, Inc.

Worden, J.W. (1991). *Grief Counseling & Grief Therapy.* New York: Springer Publishing Company.

New Initiatives Transforming Hospice Care

Stephen R. Connor

SUMMARY. Hospice care has been successful in serving a large segment of the terminally ill population in the United States. This article addresses a number of significant trends that may impact the future of hospice care. It is proposed that as many as one-third of those who die will not be in a position to make use of any end-stage program of care. Of the remaining, some will have difficulty being served by hospices due to uncertain prognosis and continued efforts at curative treatment. New models of caring for chronically terminally ill persons are being developed and are reviewed. A clearer definition of who ought to be served by hospice programs is encouraged. *[Article copies available for a fee from The Haworth Document Delivery Service: 1-800-342-9678. E-mail address: getinfo@haworthpressinc.com <Website: http://www.haworthpressinc. com>]*

INTRODUCTION

In the past twenty-five years, the hospice movement in the United States has gone from a small band of renegades to a sizable health care industry. As with other social change movements it has gone through a process of reification that has brought it from a variety of experiments to a standardized model of care. The hospice movement has been quite successful in growth, averaging an increase of 16% per year in persons served from 1985 to 1997 (NHO 1998). The National Hospice Organization reports that hospices in 1997 served approximately 495,000 terminally ill individuals and their families (NHO 1998). This represents about 20% of the 2.3 million annual deaths in the US.

[Haworth co-indexing entry note]: "New Initiatives Transforming Hospice Care." Connor, Stephen R. Co-published simultaneously in *The Hospice Journal* (The Haworth Press, Inc.) Vol. 14, No. 3/4, 1999, pp. 193-203; and: *The Hospice Heritage: Celebrating Our Future* (ed: Inge B. Corless and Zelda Foster) The Haworth Press, Inc., 1999, pp. 193-203. Single or multiple copies of this article are available for a fee from The Haworth Document Delivery Service [1-800-342-9678, 9:00 a.m. - 5:00 p.m. (EST). E-mail address: getinfo@haworthpressinc.com].

Still there are health care leaders who say that hospices are not having a large enough impact on the care of the dying; that there are still 80% of people who die who are not served by hospices. The current financing model for hospice care is based on the Medicare Hospice Benefit (MHB). Eligibility requirements for the MHB have tended to limit those who can be served by a hospice program. Most importantly patients must be certified as having six months or less to live if the disease runs its normal course and the patient must be willing to forgo further attempts at curative treatment.

As hospices have become more successful at serving those who are dying they have encountered more people who do not fit the requirements of this model. Many people are unwilling to discontinue seeking curative treatment even when the chances for effective treatment are minimal. The MHB eligibility is based on a belief that we can accurately predict six month mortality in most cases. Unfortunately we are not able to accurately predict death within six months for most individual patients. Thus there are many people who will not qualify for the MHB. In addition for anyone to make use of any kind of end-of-life program there must be some endstage to the disease or condition. For a significant number of people who die there is no endstage; there is a sudden decline and death.

An analysis of death data from the Centers for Disease Control and Prevention for 1996 (CDC 1998) reveals that there were 2,314,690 deaths from all causes. The total can be categorized into three areas; first those who died of causes which had a downhill course eventually resulting in death. These people would be appropriate for the hospice benefit as it is currently designed. Diseases include most of the malignant neoplasms, about a third of the major cardiovascular diseases, most of the chronic obstructive pulmonary diseases, some of those with late effects of cerebrovascular diseases, many of the kidney and liver disease deaths, congenital and perinatal deaths, dementias and HIV disease patients. This amounts to about 39% of total deaths.

The second group are all those who die of conditions where there is no end stage; death is sudden, after a short course of illness, or of an unpredictable condition. Included in this group are all the infectious disease deaths (non-HIV), homicides, suicides, accidents, most of the strokes, acute MIs and other non-chronic cardiovascular conditions, diabetics, and many of those where the cause of death is other or ill-defined. This group amounts to about 33% of all deaths.

There is a third group of deaths which are primarily from chronic illnesses where the course of illness is so difficult to predict that they are never labeled as end stage yet they have a condition which will result in their death. Included in this group are many of the chronic cardiovascular conditions, most of the strokes, some of the malignancies, some COPD, liver, kidney, perinatal, and other conditions. This group includes the remaining 28% of deaths.

What this means for hospice and other end-of-life care programs is that the denominator for who will use any service aimed at end-of-life care is about two-thirds of deaths! The other one third will die suddenly or won't reach a condition where they will be seen as dying or needing extensive services. So we ought to consider whether we want to stay with the current hospice model and add other services for the 28% who do not fit our model, or change the hospice model to accommodate those who we cannot now serve.

EMERGING TRENDS

In the last ten years or more, hospices have experimented with different models to expand service to patients. A significant number of patients do not qualify for the MHB due to uncertain prognosis or desire to continue attempts at curative treatment. Some hospices have used the home health agency (HHA) benefit to pay for services to patients who did not qualify for the MHB. This required them to become licensed and certified to provide HHA services. Others have provided free services to these patients using a variety of funding sources.

The primary motivation for expanding services to those who do not qualify for the MHB has been a mission driven desire to reach and serve as many dying persons as possible. Some also saw it as good business. The federal government has tended to view this as a questionable activity. Under laws prohibiting actions which encourage use of or referral for Medicare benefits (Stark I & II), providers have been warned to discontinue providing free services.

If the purpose of providing the free care was to give some consideration to another provider in return for Medicare referrals, then it violates these provisions. There have been reports of hospices in competitive markets engaging in activities that appear to be directed at encouraging referrals. For example a hospice that provides care to patients in a skilled nursing facility (SNF) through a contract may provide free care to patients who are admitted to the SNF. This is done because they qualify for skilled Medicare Part A coverage and revoke their Hospice Part A benefit to access it.

While this may encourage cooperation on the SNF's part it rarely results in a material increase in hospice's referrals. It has been done because of the hospice's desire to serve that individual until their death and not to abandon the person. It is also a considerable financial loss for the hospice program. Other free care or service may appear more questionable; for example, the hospice that stations home health aides in a SNF to care for its patients but who also delivers care to other patients in the facility.

A system that prevents providers from being able to experiment with creative ways of serving a specialized population and that sees honest community service as fraud and abuse may have gone too far. Rather than being part of the solution it has created additional problems. Although hospices need to be freed from unreasonable scrutiny and allowed to reinvent themselves to achieve their mission, there will still need to be limits which will prevent unscrupulous providers from taking advantage of the system.

Currently, there is debate over the future of the Hospice Medicare Benefit. There has been a push to revamp the MHB to address changes in the health care system which are tending to limit access to hospice services. On one side of this discussion are those who believe we should maintain the current MHB provisions. The MHB is seen as being the vehicle for hospice growth and should not be tampered with. Any changes to the MHB could open the possibility of losing the benefit.

On the other side of this debate is a realization that provisions agreed to in the early 1980s have created obstacles for the growth of hospice care beyond those patients with predictable prognoses who want only symptom-focused palliative care. The development of new treatments for cancer and prolongative therapies for chronic illnesses have put hospice in the position of forcing patients to choose between expensive and aggressive treatments that they want and receiving hospice care.

In many respects this conflict touches on the very purpose for which hospice care exists. *Is hospice only intended for those who want symptom focused treatment or is it for anyone who is facing death?* This is a fundamental question that has never been resolved by the movement. It is clear that there are people who advocate for either position. For those who believe hospice must limit itself to those who are ready to begin facing their death the answer is to maintain the current arrangement with perhaps a few minor changes.

For those who believe hospice's mission is to reach all who are facing death, major changes in the structure are required. The MHB would have to be changed in such a way that patients could receive any treatment they wished. If its effects were to prolong life that would be acceptable. The six-month limit on care would need to be changed so that anyone with a life-limiting illness would qualify. Some criteria for coverage such as severity of need would have to be substituted. A change in service delivery and payment would need to occur so that the treatment plans would be able to accommodate chronically ill patients whose courses were more variable. After an intense initial set up of services there may need to be periods of minimal care punctuated by effective response to crisis to prevent hospitalization.

Such major changes in the structure of the hospice care needs thoughtful deliberation by the field. If hospices chose to continue to serve those able to be accommodated by the current model, then growth may be limited to the approximately 39% who fit that model. If a more expansive model is embraced then the larger two-thirds or more of all deaths may be served. Clearly we need models of end-of-life care which can reach more of those who are currently suffering from life-limiting conditions.

MISSION

It may be helpful as we look to the future to go back to the beginning to address the fundamental issue of hospice's mission. Fundamentally we need to understand the core unchanging part of what makes hospice if we are to succeed. As Jim Collins (1997) has said you can change all the delivery mechanisms you want as long as you are clear on the essential core identity or ideology of your work which must never change.

Early work by the religious charities with the dying was simple enough. They tended to the gravely ill without regard to diagnosis or prognosis. In those days the science was limited and one rarely knew what was causing the person to fail other than God's will. This was a model primarily based on severity of need. The focus of care was on the basic necessities of food, water, and cleanliness. Patients suffered due to the lack of knowledge of palliative care and the lack of effective medications.

This situation changed when the founder of the modern hospice movement, Dame Cicely Saunders, established the science of palliative medicine. Attention to the whole person and family coupled with scientific rigor in developing effective treatment for pain and symptoms were the building blocks of the modern hospice movement.

Dame Saunders noted that hospice care is not for everyone who is dying; it is for a portion of the dying who have a relatively progressive and predictable demise. Dame Saunders feels that other specialists are better prepared to care for the other non-cancer terminal illnesses (personal communication). Others in the UK are interested in seeing hospice expand to serve a larger proportion of those dying of chronic illness. In her initial policies for admission at St. Christopher's Hospice only those with predictable progressive terminal illness were admitted. This was effectively those with metastatic cancers and those with motor neuron disease such as Lou Gehrig's Disease (Amyotrophic Lateral Sclerosis). Until recently those with chronic terminal illnesses such as congestive heart failure, chronic obstructive pulmonary disease, dementia, and so forth, were not eligible for admission.

In the US the hospice movement began with a broad interest in the experience of dying. It began in the context of a consumer movement that was trying to engage the public in being more involved in health and treatment of illness. There were no insurance benefits and those involved volunteered their time in the service of humanizing the care of the terminally ill. There was little structure other than those broad principles imported from St. Christopher's Hospice in England.

The US hospice movement veered away from institutionally based care to a home care model with the development of the Medicare Hospice Benefit. American independence and consumer orientation put high value on being in one's home and hearth when death neared and government officials, concerned with a new program that could add to the costs of care, emphasized home care. Without insurance limitations and the risks of managed care, some hospices served all those who came their way even when chemotherapy or other treatment continued. Hospice providers walked the journey with the patient and family and supported them in the decisions they made. With few effective treatments available, patients and families eventually elected a palliative care approach.

Given the current limitations hospices are experiencing it might be tempting to suggest that we simply return to the early days of hospice in the US with all of its flexibility and volunteerism. However, if there had been no hospice benefit, the movement today would constitute a small ineffective fringe activity in the health care system and could truly be dismissed as irrelevant. What these benefits have brought and bought are an extensive array of real services delivered to enormous numbers of real people who are dying.

The dilemma is that patients cannot now have the support of hospice and continue an aggressive search for effective treatment for their life threatening conditions. This brings us back to the central question of who are hospice's patients? Not all chronically ill persons will need the extensive services of a hospice team. The real target population for hospice and end-of-life care programs are those whose disease severity and life disruption is so great that they will need specialized help in living with their illness. These are usually desperately ill patients who will die soon or will continue to undergo a roller coaster of ups and downs in their illness.

EMERGING MODELS

A number of emerging models of end-of-life care will have considerable impact on hospice care. They include the palliative care model, the Medicaring model, and the disease/case/care management model. While they have aspects in common I will focus on each individually, identifying their differences.

The *palliative care* model harks back to some of the early structures tried when hospice care was beginning. Most of the current palliative care programs are hospital based programs. They usually involve the formation of a palliative care team, headed by a physician, who intervenes in the care of patients throughout an institution who are having symptom management problems. Many have developed inpatient palliative care units for intense symptom management. Some palliative care programs have developed along side hospice programs. They function to serve those terminally ill persons who are not eligible for hospice care who want to continue aggressive chemotherapy or do not want to enter hospice for psychological reasons.

An early example of a palliative care team was the hospice program at St. Luke's hospital in New York City. This program used a mobile interdisciplinary team to assist dying patients in all parts of the hospital. It was funded by the hospital but never had its own unique source of reimbursement and finally stopped operation. A current palliative care team operates out of the Cleveland Clinic under the direction of Dr. Declan Walsh. This palliative care program continues aggressive chemotherapy for its terminally ill cancer patients while using other symptom management options. Only those patients who do not want chemotherapy are admitted to the hospice program.

The *Medicaring* Program being developed by Dr. Joanne Lynn at the Center to Improve Care of the Dying is an effort to develop a continuing care model for congestive heart failure and chronic obstructive pulmonary disease patients. This program is in the process of being tested in a number of sites that include the VA system and a variety of hospice programs. Patients eligible for participation in Medicaring include those with life expectancies of 1-2 years. Two hospitalizations in the year prior to admission qualifies them for participation. They receive a comprehensive assessment and a variety of services designed to optimally treat their condition. The goal is a more stable disease course with fewer exacerbations. The program evaluation is being designed and will attempt to demonstrate cost effectiveness by effectively reducing hospitalizations.

Medicaring is one example of attempts to manage more effectively particularly difficult disease states. *Disease state management* programs being developed attempt to prevent exacerbations of disease from occurring to such an extent that they require hospitalization. These programs range from treatment of asthma and diabetes to cancer and heart disease.

Care or case management programs develop methods for managing the care of patients with severe illnesses. Again the aim is to keep the patient in a stabilized condition thus improving health care and minimizing cost. Emphasis is on education of the patient and family in optimal care and provision of services based on need at different points in the illness trajectory. Effective case management ability in the population of gravely ill or dying persons requires the ability to respond to the needs of patients face to face. Like hospice care there has to be the ability to respond to a patient at 2 a.m. if necessary to prevent a hospitalization.

With life limiting illnesses it would make more sense to have a plan for treatment of the patient which begins at diagnosis and ends at death. Palliative treatment would be available at many points in the continuum. Specialized and more intensive palliative care (hospice) would be available during the end stage of the illness. It remains unclear how effective the medical system can be in dealing with the reality of patient dying. A specialized program of care for dying patients may always be needed.

Using the various possible trajectories we have discussed earlier we can see (see Figure 1) that there are several general scenarios which occur:

1. Those who die suddenly or after a short course of illness (MI, infectious disease, etc.);
2. Those who die of a predictable downhill course of illness (cancer, ALS, etc.);
3. Those who die of a chronic illness with exacerbations who convert to a more predictable course under palliative management; and
4. Those with chronic illness who continue with intermittent exacerbations until a final difficult to predict demise.

FUTURE SCENARIOS

The attempt to improve end-of-life care in the U.S. may unfold in a number of ways. First there could be a restructuring of the Medicare Hospice Benefit in such a way that more dying patients could be served. This would involve expanding eligibility requirements to allow admission of terminally ill persons with greater than a six-month prognosis or without a prognostic requirement, different payment provisions based on severity of illness and length of stay, and reduction of risk for high cost elements of care.

A second scenario could involve keeping the current Medicare Hospice Benefit conditions of participation and creation of another service mechanism to provide care to those who are not appropriate for the current benefit but who will need enhanced services. This could be through provision of a palliative care or case management program for those with severe conditions that would eventually result in death.

FIGURE 1. Varying Trajectories of Dying

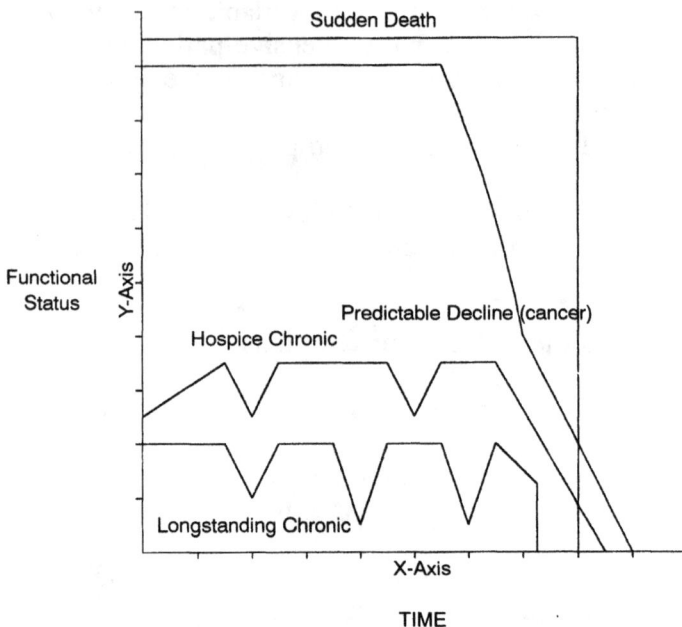

Unfortunately there are other scenarios where there is no improvement or a decline in the quality of end-of-life care. There is some concern that opening the door to any changes to the Medicare Hospice Benefit could result in a step backwards. The MHB is really an extraordinary benefit that is unprecedented. It allows for an unusual amount of autonomy for hospice providers and in spite of it's limitations has had a major impact on care at the end-of-life in the US.

There is currently a great deal of interest in care at the end-of-life. Two major factors are driving this interest, the acknowledgement by the medical establishment that care of the dying is poor coupled with a growing public interest in physician-assisted suicide. This interest and opportunity to improve care for the dying may eventually wane. It is important that this opportunity not be lost. A vigorous dialogue among those who care for the dying is needed. Improvements in how our systems of care work can be made. What we must not do is to lose ground in the advances we have made. Changing the system so that fewer people use hospice care appropriately would be a step backwards. We must add more options for care of the sickest.

DISCUSSION

We have examined the emergence of hospice care in the US and how the Medicare Hospice Benefit has fueled the growth of a new type of provider focused exclusively on the care of dying persons. The details of mortality data have been examined revealing that as many as a third of those who die in the US will never be in a position to use hospice or any end-of-life care program due to the circumstances and trajectory of their conditions. Also noted are the limitations of the current hospice payment system which exclude many of those who are in need of extensive services in their final months. This realization has brought into focus the need to reexamine the mission of hospice and to further clarify who ought to be served by a hospice program.

A variety of additional new models of care for chronically, terminally ill persons are being proposed and are examined. It remains to be seen whether hospice care ought to be expanded to include a broader range of people who die or whether new models of care delivery distinct from hospice care ought to be supported.

There is much at stake in this discussion. The future of a largely successful movement to improve care of the dying hangs in the balance. So to do the lives and deaths of hundreds of thousands of Americans each year.

REFERENCES

Center for Disease Control and Prevention (November 10, 1998). *National Vital Statistics Reports for 1996.* Vol. 47 (9).

Collins, James & Porras, Jerry (1994). *Built to last: Successful habits of visionary companies.* Harpercollins.

National Hospice Organization (1997). *Results of National Hospice Census for 1995.* Arlington, VA: NHO.

National Hospice Organization (1998). *Fact Sheet from the National Hospice Organization.* Arlington, VA: NHO.

Personal communication with Dame Cicely Saunders, Nov. 25, 1996.

REFLECTIONS AND REMINISCENCES

Reflections on Death in America

George Soros

SUMMARY. The project on Death in America was established to promote a better understanding of the experience of dying and bereavement and by doing so help transform the culture surrounding death. The Faculty Scholars Program provides three year fellowships for projects that explore critical aspects of the care of the dying, for those who will become academic leaders on the issue, as well as, role models and mentors to future generations of health professionals. A Grants Program broad enough to cover every aspect of the culture of dying allocates funding for innovative projects. A new grants program is underway to support projects aimed at enhancing the role of the humanities in transforming the culture of death and dying in America. *[Article copies available for a fee from The Haworth Document Delivery Service: 1-800-342-9678. E-mail address: getinfo@haworthpressinc.com <Website: http://www.haworthpressinc.com>]*

KEYWORDS. Project on Death in America, PDLA, faculty scholars, death

---

Printed with permission from Michael Vachon, Director of Communications, Open Society Institute.

This article is an adaptation from a speech at the College of Physicians and Surgeons at Columbia University in November 1994 soon after the establishment of the Project on Death in America.

[Haworth co-indexing entry note]: "Reflections on Death in America." Soros, George. Co-published simultaneously in *The Hospice Journal* (The Haworth Press, Inc.) Vol. 14, No. 3/4, 1999, pp. 205-215; and: *The Hospice Heritage: Celebrating Our Future* (ed: Inge B. Corless and Zelda Foster) The Haworth Press, Inc., 1999, pp. 205-215.

The Project on Death in America was established four years ago. The mission of the Project is to promote a better understanding of the experience of dying and bereavement and by doing so help transform the culture surrounding death. To do this, the Project set out to support initiatives in research, scholarship, the humanities and the arts, as well as innovations in the provision of care, public education, professional education, and public policy. My personal hope is for the ratio between research and action to be heavily weighed toward action. Initially, I committed five million dollars a year to the Project's work for three years and recently approved the same amount of support for another three years. I sponsored the Project for two reasons: one very abstract, the other very personal.

The abstract motivation derives from a basic insight which has been at the root of both my money-making and my philanthropic activities and which I have elaborated into a not-yet-properly-understood philosophical theory. The insight is that there is always a divergence between the views and ideas that guide people in their actions and the actual state of affairs. I call the divergence the "participant's bias." Since the participant's actions help shape reality, there is a two-way feedback mechanism between the participant's bias and the events in which they participate. I call this two-way feedback "reflexivity."

Sometimes the participant's bias is quite small and there are forces at play which tend to bring the participant's views and the actual state of affairs closer together. But at other times the bias can be quite enormous without any tendency to correct itself. On the contrary, the two-way feedback mechanism may help validate and reinforce the bias until the situation becomes untenable and there is a reversal in the self-reinforcing process.

Everybody has experienced such far-from-equilibrium situations in his life, but I have specialized in them. I lived through Nazi persecution in Hungary as an adolescent, then I had a taste of communism and when I went to England I came under the influence of Karl Popper, the philosopher of science, and began to develop my theory of reflexivity. When I became involved in the financial markets I specialized on boom/bust sequences and did rather well out of them. And when I made more money than I could use for my personal needs I set up a foundation devoted to the idea of an open society. Without going too deeply into it, open society is based on the principle that we all act on imperfect knowledge and nobody is in possession of the ultimate truth.

A society based on the recognition that we may be wrong is preferable to a society which denies that its leaders may be wrong.

I set up foundations which tried to help open up closed societies and I became rather intimately involved in the revolutionary process which led from one kind of far-from-equilibrium situation to another; from the rigidity of the Soviet system to the chaos of its collapse. In the first five years, following the fall of communism, I was very busy because one can do many things in the heat of the revolutionary moment which would be impossible in normal times. But as the revolution began to cool off I began to think what I could do to make our own open society more viable; because according to my theory, open societies also suffer from deficiencies which need to be recognized and corrected for open societies to remain viable. Initially, I focused on two problem areas where misconceptions play a particularly important role, making the problems worse than they would be if they were better understood. One is the problem of dying. The other is the problem of drugs where the remedy is worse than the disease.

Due to our imperfect understanding, our actions have unintended consequences. Nowhere are they more glaring than in the war on drugs. By treating drug abuse as a crime, we have created crime, corruption, and violence which are much more destructive than drug abuse by itself. I should like to see the false identifications between drug and crime broken without necessarily advocating the legalization of drugs. These both have one thing in common: distortions and misconceptions aggravate the problem. I chose the problem of dying because of some very personal experiences in connection with the death of my parents, both of whom I was very devoted to and loved dearly.

My father died at home in 1963. He was terminally ill. Although he agreed to an operation, he didn't particularly want to survive it because he was afraid that the combination of the illness and the operation would invade and destroy his autonomy as a human being. Unfortunately, that in fact is what happened. After the operation he had very little time left. I'm afraid I kind of wrote him off at the point. I was there when he died, yet I let him die alone. I could see him, but I wasn't at his bedside. The day after he died I went into the office. I didn't talk about my father's death. So I kind of denied his dying, I certainly didn't participate in it. Afterwards, I read Kubler-Ross and learned that I might have maintained contact with him if I tried. Had I read Kubler-Ross earlier I would have probably held his hand, because I did love him. I just didn't know that it might make a difference. I forgave myself because I did not know any better.

My mother's death was more recent. She had joined the Hemlock Society and had at hand a means of doing away with herself. I asked her if she needed my help; I offered it, although I wasn't particularly keen to do it. But I would have helped her because I felt that I owed it to her. At the point of decision, however, she did not want to take her own life, and I'm glad she didn't. Her decision gave the family a chance to rally around and be there as she prepared to die. And this time we did maintain good contact right to the end.

She had this experience, which is described in Kubler-Ross, of walking up to the gates of heaven, and I was accompanying her. She told me she was worried that she might drag me with her. So I reassured her that I was firmly ensconced on this earth and she should not worry. Her dying was really a very positive experience for all of us because of the way she handled herself and the way the family, not just me but particularly my children, could participate in it.

These two personal experiences made me realize that there is a need to better understand the experience of dying. In my initial research in the issue I was assisted by a friend, Patricia Prem, who as a social worker had dealt professionally with dying. She brought together the people who helped create the Project on Death in America. She is on the Project's advisory board now, as are:

- *Susan Block*, Harvard Medical School
- *Robert Burt*, Yale Law School
- *Robert Butler*, International Longevity Center
- *David Rothman*, Columbia College of Physicians and Surgeons
- *William D. Zabel*, Attorney
- *Kathleen M. Foley*, Chief of the Pain and Palliative Care Service at the Sloan-Kettering Memorial Cancer Center and Director of the Project on Death in America

Now, let us look briefly at what we want to transform and why. We will begin with a small matter, the name of our project. It took a considerable amount of discussion to rid ourselves of clever euphemisms and settle on a name that states our purpose directly, even starkly: the Project on Death in America. In America, the land of the perpetually young, growing older is an embarrassment, and dying is a failure. Death has replaced sex as the taboo subject of our times. People compete to appear on talk shows to discuss the most intimate details of their sex lives, but they have nothing to say about dying, which in its immensity dwarfs the momentary pleasures of sex. Only our preoccupation with violence breaks through this shroud of silence. Killing yes; dying no.

Even doctors, especially doctors, don't like to think about death. It is easier to find descriptions of the way people die and what can be done to ease their death in the medical textbooks of the turn-of-the-century than in today's voluminous literature on the treatment and cure of diseases.

This emphasis on treating disease, instead of providing care, has altered the practice of medicine. People live longer, surviving four or five illnesses before dying. But the health care bill grows with every illness. Our success has also brought other unintended consequences. We have created a medical culture that is so intent on curing disease and prolonging life that it fails to provide support in that inevitable phase of life–death. Advances in high technology interventions have contributed to this weakness in our medical system, deluding doctors and patients alike into believing that the inevitable can be delayed almost indefinitely.

The reality of death and the perceptions of the participants–the dying person, the doctor, the family members–are separated by a wide gap. We need to bring the two into closer alignment. Doctors who are on a first-name basis with disease must re-acquaint themselves with the patient. They must recognize that, by focusing exclusively on conquering disease and prolonging life, they abandon the dying when, in their own words, there is "nothing more to be done." They must come to terms with their own death in order to provide proper care for the dying.

Sixty-three percent of people die in hospitals, yet, for most people, hospitals are not a good place to die. Hospitals are set up to take care of acute illnesses, and dying is not an illness. It doesn't belong to an official medical category, it has no DRG (disease related category) that would permit reimbursement for the hospital and the physician. If you go to a hospital to die, the doctors have to find something wrong with you, something to treat, like pneumonia or dehydration, or they cannot admit you. They hook you up to tubes and machines and try to fix a condition that isn't fixable. The need to arrive at a reimbursable diag-

nosis changes the reality. The doctors and nurses are working to prolong life, instead of preparing a patient for death. The ideal of a
peaceful death is impossible in such an alien setting, under such extreme conditions.

A peaceful death is more likely to be achieved at home in familiar
surroundings that are more conducive to the comfort and ritual of
leave taking from family and friends. Both my parents died at home.
In my mother's case, after I accompanied her to the gates of heaven
and left her in good hands, she lost consciousness and lingered for
another seven to ten days before dying. I visited her regularly to see if
there was any sign of communication or consciousness, but there
wasn't. She died at home, because we could afford to keep her there
with round-the-clock nurses attending to her. We weren't forced by
lack of financial resources to put her into a hospital where medical
intervention may well have kept her much longer in a state of limbo
between living and dying. Just by giving her food, the process could
have been unnecessarily prolonged.

Only twenty percent of people die in their own home, a nursing
home, or a hospice. Hospices offer the kind of palliative care that
should be routine procedure in every institution that cares for the
dying. Proper care includes the control of pain and other symptoms as
well as attention to the psychological and spiritual needs of the patient.
To provide this care, hospices employ teams of doctors, nurses, social
workers, and bereavement counselors. But the hospice alternative,
unfortunately, is not available to the majority of dying patients. Medicare coverage is limited. As a result, most hospice programs deliver
care to the dying in their own home, but are restricted financially from
providing intensive custodial care. This requires the presence of a
family member who doesn't work, who is physically able, and who is
willing to assume the responsibilities for care the rest of the time.

The recommendations that follow from these observations are obvious. First and foremost, doctors, nurses, and other health professionals need better training in the care of the dying, especially in the relief
of pain. Health professionals also need training in alleviating the psychological, emotional, and existential suffering that may accompany
dying. Physical pain is what people fear most about dying. A dying
person in pain cannot think about anything else, leaving no room for
coming to terms with death, for reviewing one's life, putting one's
affairs in order, for saying goodbye. Therefore, pain relief must come

first. Doctors often undermedicate their dying patients for fear of turning them into drug addicts.

The first major program established by the Project's board was the Faculty Scholars Program. The Project selects outstanding faculty and clinicians who are committed to the Project's goals and supports them in their work of developing new models for the care of the dying and new approaches to the education of health professionals about the care of dying patients and their families. The scholars, who receive two- to three-year fellowships for projects that explore critical aspects of the care of the dying, will become the academic leaders on the issue, as well as role models and mentors to future generations of health professionals. Each year the project selects eight to ten faculty scholars. With the announcement of the fourth cohort of scholars, the Project now has leaders and role models in 33 of the country's 125 medical schools, two nursing schools and four Canadian medical schools.

The board then established a Grants Program broad enough to cover every aspect of the culture of dying including epidemiology, ethnography, and history of dying and bereavement; new service-delivery models for the dying and their family and friends; separate educational programs for the public and the health care professionals; and the shaping of governmental and institutional policy. At the end of the third year, 88 grants were funded.

Among the projects of the faculty scholars three are focused on the psychiatric aspects of end-of-life care; one on end-of-life care among chronically ill children and their families; five on new service-delivery systems for the dying and their families; and six on programs related to physician education about end-of-life issues, including pain management. Other projects include one focused on emotional and spiritual suffering among the dying; three focus on quality-improvement projects related to end-of-life care; an examination of end-of-life care practices in managed care; a study of the cost effectiveness and efficacy of end-of-life care; and a project on quality of end-of-life care measurement.

We also must increase the availability of hospice services for terminally ill patients removing restrictions on admittance and enhancing reimbursement regulations. We should consider laws that permit next of kin to decide to forego life sustaining medical interventions even when a patient's wishes are not known. Aggressive, life-prolonging interventions, which may at times go against the patient's wishes, are much more expensive than proper care for the dying. The government may have to help family members financially so that they can take care of dying persons at home by the least expensive means.

Promoting and developing hospice or palliative care was the focus of a large number of the close to 2,000 requests for grants that the Project received, as well as the 88 programs selected for funding. Three hospice grants went to support the care of dying homeless men and women in special homes in Washington, DC and Cleveland, Ohio. By creating respectful communities and hospice care, these programs serve as models for end-of-life care for vulnerable populations. They demonstrate the need for better reimbursement programs to prevent the marginalization of the dying poor.

Hospitals must be required to develop and adopt a comprehensive DRG for terminal care. This single change would go a long ways toward removing the hypocrisy that now surrounds a hospital's treatment of the dying and freeing doctors and nurses to provide the kind of care that doesn't rely on technology–such as the simple act of paying attention to a dying person, holding their hand, listening, and comforting them.

The Project supported the work of the National Committee on Financing Care at the End of Life in their work to create a DRG for payment for terminal care services delivered to hospital patients. The program will also train hospital coding administrators and other health care providers on the implementation of the code.

Can we afford to care for the dying properly? These are the questions we must ask ourselves given that the number of people dying in the United States currently stands at 2.4 million annually. Increases in cancer and AIDS deaths and the aging of the baby boomers will cause this figure to climb faster than the population. Today 1 in 8 Americans is 65 years or older. In 30 to 40 years, 1 in 5 will be in that age group. The average life expectancy for those reaching age 65 is already 81 for men and 85 for women. The fear is that the dying of the elderly will drain the national treasury. Like most fears, this one is based on a myth, the popular perception that elderly, terminally ill patients consume enormous amounts of resources shortly before they die.

It is true that nearly half of all medical expenses are incurred in the last six months of people's lives. But it is also true that medical expenditures in the last year of life are lower for people 80 years and older than for those in younger age groups. *Seven Deadly Myths:*

Uncovering the Facts About the High Cost of the Last Year of Life, a report produced by the Alliance for Aging Research with the Project's support, elaborates on the myths that have been created from faulty common assumptions and offers recommendations in response to the actual state of affairs.

In *Approaching Death: Improving Care at the End of Life,* a book-length report published in September 1997 and funded by the Project, the Institute of Medicine examined the state of knowledge about clinical, behavioral, legal, economic, and other important aspects of care for patients with life-threatening medical problems; evaluated methods for measuring outcomes and assessing quality of care; identified factors that impede or promote high quality care for patients approaching death; and recommended steps that policymakers, practitioners, and others could take to improve care. The report is likely to serve as a tremendous resource as communities nation-wide grapple with better ways to care for the dying.

The one aspect of dying that is talked about everywhere–on television, in public forums, in newspaper headlines, and serious journal articles–is physician-assisted suicide and euthanasia. In October 1997 voters in Oregon approved, for the second time, a law allowing physician-assisted suicide. It is the first state to take this step.

As the son of a mother who was a member of the Hemlock Society, and as a reader of Plato's *Phaedra,* I cannot but approve. But I must emphasize that I am speaking in my personal capacity and not on behalf of the Board of the Project on Death in America. In 1997, the Project filed an amicus brief in the two Supreme Court cases concerning physician-assisted suicide, arguing that the Court should not find a constitutional right to such assistance until we, as a society, have taken measures to assure that the terminally ill who consider suicide are not motivated by the failure of doctors to treat their pain or depression, or by economic fears.

As founder of the project, I respect their judgement. I believe in personal autonomy; I believe people should be allowed to determine their own end. But I also recognize that legalizing euthanasia could have unintended consequences, leading to all kind of abuses. The issues need to be carefully weighed, but I accept that this is not the first priority of the Project. Very few terminally ill patients would avail themselves of the opportunity, even if euthanasia were legalized. After all, my mother refused my help and I am glad she did. The Project on

Death in America concerns itself with the vast majority of people who are not looking for physician-assisted suicide and they have their work cut out for them.

In its second three years, the Project will focus its efforts on several major initiatives while maintaining a commitment to health care professional education and training. The Project plans to engage the major professional associations for nursing, social work and pastoral care in end-of-life care issues and to support their efforts to develop innovative approaches to field specific education, training, and research on these issues. A new grants program is underway to support projects aimed at enhancing the role of the humanities in transforming the culture of death and dying in America. In response to the dearth of data on the financing of care at the end of life, the Project convened a meeting of health economists and other experts to identify the areas ripe for research and develop strategies for reducing identifiable economic barriers to quality care at life's end. Another initiative will explore the advantages and disadvantages of using litigation to address state and federal legal barriers to adequate care at the end of life. The Project's new de Tocqueville Enterprise funding initiative will support grassroots, community-based efforts to link professional and volunteer care-taking organizations within several communities around the United States.

Grantmakers Concerned with Care at the End of Life is a coalition of funders who came together to support and promote the vital role of the philanthropic community in transforming and improving the care of the dying. The Project was a founding member of the coalition and in the coming years will support the expansion of GCCEL's membership and continued efforts to educate funders on end-of-life issues.

The Project will continue its efforts to share the knowledge its grantees have gathered and the models that have been developed with health care professionals and the public through a variety of forums including conferences, the Website and PDIA Newsletter. For example, the Project co-hosted a national conference with the Open Society Institute's Center on Crime, Community and Culture on care of the dying in prisons and jails.

In conclusion, let me tell you how I came to terms with my own death–a subject I gave a lot of thought to in my youth. I spent years thinking about it. Building on my insight that there is always a divergence between ideas and facts I came to the conclusion that it is the idea of my own death which I cannot accept because it is a total denial of my consciousness. The fact of dying, when it comes, may be much more acceptable, especially if it comes at the end of a long life. The insight that the idea is not the same as the fact, made the idea more bearable.

I am sure that I would not find the argument persuasive if I had to confront the fact of my death here and now but as an idea I find it both convincing and comforting. I wonder whether it has the same effect on you when you hear it for the first time.

Personal Reflections

Claire B. Tehan

SUMMARY. A hospice pioneer and veteran of 23 years reflects on the early days of the hospice movement in the United States. The political, social and economic forces, which shaped the industry, are addressed from a local state and national perspective. Current challenges are briefly referenced with a call for hospice leaders to recognize the need for and identify where hospice fits into the broad end of life discussions. *[Article copies available for a fee from The Haworth Document Delivery Service: 1-800-342-9678. E-mail address: getinfo@haworthpressinc.com <Website: http://www.haworthpressinc.com>]*

KEYWORDS. Terminally ill patient, end of life, National Hospice Organization, California State Hospice Association, Medicare hospice benefit, palliative care, hospice standards, Hospice Demonstration Project

> *Time present and time past*
> *Are both perhaps present in time future*
> *And time future contained in time past.*
>
> T. S. Eliot

I appreciate the opportunity to reflect on my 23 years of involvement in hospice. While I have spent virtually my entire professional life in one field, I can say that the experience has never been static. These past 23 years has been an evolution: the program in California

---

[Haworth co-indexing entry note]: "Personal Reflections." Tehan, Claire B. Co-published simultaneously in *The Hospice Journal* (The Haworth Press, Inc.) Vol. 14, No. 3/4, 1999, pp. 217-228; and: *The Hospice Heritage: Celebrating Our Future* (ed: Inge B. Corless and Zelda Foster) The Haworth Press, Inc., 1999, pp. 217-228. Single or multiple copies of this article are available for a fee from The Haworth Document Delivery Service [1-800-342-9678, 9:00 a.m. - 5:00 p.m. (EST). E-mail address: getinfo@haworthpressinc. com].

that I initiated in 1977 has evolved from serving 78 patients the first year to becoming one of the initial 26 HCFA Hospice Demonstration Projects. Thereafter the program became a Medicare certified hospice, and is now a multi-site regional hospice provider which provides hospice care to over 1,500 patients and families each year. Simultaneously, I have served in multiple leadership positions in California and on the national level. My reflections, therefore, reflect the dual role as a provider and as someone involved in policy issues at the state and national levels. The opportunity to participate at those levels has added a breadth and depth to my management skills, has enriched our program and my personal and professional life.

I have had the opportunity to be part of a movement from inception through its stages of infancy, growth and acceptance as a legitimate part of the health care system. My introduction to hospice began in 1972 as a UCLA graduate student when I tackled the issue of physician attitudes towards euthanasia for my Master's thesis. Two years later, a Rochester, New York oncologist asked me to develop a hospice program at the University of Rochester Cancer Center. I was young, enthusiastic and naive to the politics of university teaching hospitals and jumped at the opportunity.

It actually didn't take that long to figure out that a hospice program as part of the continuum of care at the Cancer Center was too threatening to a system focused on research and aggressive treatment. However, I personally benefited from the chance to be involved in the American hospice movement from the beginning. In 1976, I spent time with Florence Wald at the Connecticut Hospice, which had developed a hospice home care program, with plans to build a free standing hospice facility. I also spent time with Dr. Balfour Mount at The Royal Victoria Hospital in Montreal who introduced me to the Canadian approach, which included a Palliative Care Unit as the base of operations supplemented by a small home care team. I also traveled to "Mecca"–St. Christopher's Hospice in England. My three weeks on site included the opportunity to be with Dr. Cicely Saunders, the founder of the modern hospice movement, and a woman who let no obstacle stand in her way in creating a model approach to care of the dying. When the trip was arranged, no one had specifically inquired as to my professional background. I did not fit into their usual clinical program for nurses, social workers, or chaplain, so they created an internship on the spot. It meant that I had a chance to observe all aspects of the program–the facility itself, the home care program, the administration, the bereavement program. What I learned was that St. Christopher's did what they said–provided expert and humane care to terminally ill patients–and they were every bit as good as I had hoped.

These opportunities to learn about the earliest hospice program in the United States, Canada and England were undertaken on behalf of the Cancer Center which was not yet ready to implement a hospice program. However, by 1977, I had returned to Los Angeles with a vision of hospice care that was inspired by my interactions with these pioneers and my observations of their programs. I was extremely fortunate to meet Kaye Daniels, founder of Hospital Home Health Care Agency of California (HHHCA) and to be given the chance, by her, to develop the Hospice Program. She had faith that I could guide and develop a quality hospice home care program, even though I was not a registered nurse. She recognized that hospice care goes beyond the traditional medical model and that my perspective, unencumbered by a nursing or social work bias and tempered by my course work in public health, would result in an organizational approach designed to meet the needs of patients, families and hospitals in Los Angeles. It seems strange now, but in 1977, it was very unusual for someone who was not a nurse to be a hospice director. I learned a tremendous amount from Kaye and the early success of our program is due in large part to her guidance and support.

HOSPICE LEADERSHIP

The mood of hospice leaders in the 1970s was what you would expect from crusaders; the energy and enthusiasm for improving care of the dying was seemingly boundless. We were crusaders, visionaries–people committed to changing the way people lived and died. The inadequacies of the health care system in caring for terminally ill patients were the springboard for our action. From every corner of the country and every discipline, leaders emerged: Dan Hadlock, Ed Olsen, Dorothy Moga, Bob Canny, Beau Bohart, Bill Lamers, Sandol Stoddard, Mary Taverna, Gary Jacobsen, Rev. Bill Manger, Charlotte Shedd, Ina Ajemian, Bernice Harper, Carmian Seifert, Karen Sobeck, Anne Katterhagen, Peter Keese, Mary Cummings, and Dick Brett, to name just a few!

We were amazingly naive–naive to the resistance from the medical community. It was inconceivable that physicians wouldn't see the value and worth of hospice. Somehow, the fact that Dr. Elizabeth Kubler-Ross, a pioneer in the field, had been rebuffed by physicians at University of Chicago Medical Center in her request to interview terminally ill patients for her groundbreaking book, *On Death and Dying,* did not register with us.

We simply did not believe that physicians in our local hospitals would deny having any terminally ill patients. Of course, we could help them improve the care of their patients! Their initial response was to dismiss our symptom management skills and to compliment our "hand holding" abilities. Our approach to pain control, which included anticipating and preventing pain, as well as the use of round the clock administration of narcotics, was met with considerable resistance by many physicians and nurses. Hospice's recognition of the need to address psychological, spiritual and emotional pain was frequently discounted.

While progress in converting the medical community was slow, our efforts at public education were quite different. Almost everyone knew someone with cancer who had suffered excruciating pain and thus could relate to our holistic approach to pain management. The concept of care inclusive of all family members struck a responsive chord in the public. We were busy with public speaking engagements and it was easy to gain media attention. Human interest stories in newspapers, on radio, and television were part of every hospice's public education campaign. Contrary to today's emphasis on rooting out "fraud and abuse," the media fell all over itself to explain the hospice concept. The excitement of creating a new model of care for dying patients generated a momentum that carried us forward. The responsiveness of the public, and the patients and families we cared for, sustained us as we tried to convert the medical community.

Nurses, social workers, psychologists, volunteers, and graduate students came flocking to our programs. There was no shortage of people who wanted to get involved, who wanted to be part of this new humanistic movement. One of the most valuable and lasting impacts of hospice has been the training programs for hospice volunteers throughout the country. In our program, volunteers committed to 30-40 hours of training, as well as one year of service. As members of the interdisciplinary team, we prepared them thoroughly for we knew they had to function as part of our professional staff. Many hospice programs relied exclusively on volunteers for their professional services. Across the country, a grass roots movement of lay and professional volunteers, knowledgeable and thoroughly schooled in the hospice philosophy of care, developed. It is fair to say that almost everyone who completed these trainings described it as a life transforming experience. Regardless of the number of years a hospice volunteer provides service, the knowledge and insights gained from the training last a lifetime.

This grass roots momentum not only fueled the pioneers–to work tirelessly in our own communities to build effective and viable programs–but also to leap into a larger arena, the state or national level. It didn't take long to recognize that we could broaden access to hospice care for terminally ill patients only by working together to effect more change, create policy, and work for coverage of hospice care by insurance companies. Hospice programs were so poor that hiring staff to lobby or present our case to regulators was simply not an option. Many programs felt fortunate to have enough funds to attend conferences related to hospice care. My initial involvement began with the Southern California Hospice Association (which later became the California State Hospice Association), which brought together hospice leaders from Santa Barbara to San Diego. I subsequently became involved on a national level with the National Hospice Organization. It is difficult to decide which aspects of the early years to spotlight but the snapshots of a few memorable moments and some of the early organizational work will comprise my view of the landscape.

In California, two separate regional organizations, the Bay Area Hospice Association and the Southern California Hospice Association, were formed. With virtually no money but considerable dedication and commitment, these organizations significantly advanced the development of hospice care. Early state leaders included Dr. Pierre Salmon, Charles Zimmer, Larry Beresford, Sarah Gorodezky, Barbara Noggle, Mary Taverna, Donna Spaulding, Doug McKrell, and Betty Wood. In Southern California, we realized significant benefits from sharing ideas, approaches and expertise with each other. We were all unbelievably generous with our knowledge, sharing policies, procedures, brochures, marketing materials and forms, etc., which we had individually developed. There was virtually no sense of competitiveness in the early years, because the area was so vast, the resources so limited, the obstacles so many and the enormity of the task, to change the culture of dying, so daunting.

Given the infamous "divide" between Northern and Southern California, the two organizations accomplished the unthinkable, years later, and merged into the California State Hospice Association. When I served as the elected President of that organization for three years, all of the materials related to that organization fit in one corner of my office. Today, the Sacramento based organization employs a paid executive director and staff and has proven its effectiveness in representing the interests of hospice providers in California. The California State Hospice Association is a unifying force in the state and was a critical factor in winning the eleven-year battle for hospice licensure. Similar experiences have been repeated in many states.

In 1977, I attended the first organizing meeting of the National Hospice Organization in Branford, Connecticut. Dennis Rezendez of The Connecticut Hospice, and Zachary Morfogen of The Riverside Hospice in Morristown, New Jersey were instrumental in establishing the National Hospice Organization. Their vision, political, organizational and fundraising savvy was critical to this national effort.

One of the first committees developed by NHO was the Standards and Accreditation Committee. I volunteered for that committee because like the other committee members we had a vision of hospice care that would include hospices in every state. We recognized that 57 varieties of hospice care would lead to public confusion as to what hospice care really was. And that was the status of hospice care at the time. Hospice was local . . . and reflected each community that it served. This was its strength and its success–and a huge weakness in the effort to truly broaden access, for there was no guarantee that essential services were offered. For example, even though the interdisciplinary team was a fundamental component of hospice, some programs relied almost exclusively on psychosocial caregivers with little nursing intervention. The converse was also true, there was nursing care with no additional psychosocial support.

The Standards and Accreditation Committee included representatives from North Carolina, Connecticut, Delaware, Minnesota, California, and Missouri. We all recognized that shared values were not sufficient for establishing credibility for the hospice movement and that only the development of national standards would provide a uniform definition of hospice care. We also knew that we needed to clearly identify the essential values and basic components of hospice care, in order to protect the public.

I still remember the hue and cry from hospice providers around the country–How could we? How dare we try and tell anyone how to provide hospice care? Providers, particularly those with all-volunteer models, were outraged that a bureaucratic definition of hospice was being instituted. Some people saw the development of national standards as unnecessary, unfair, and the ultimate ruination of this "pure" movement. Those of us who "signed up" to develop the NHO standards–and many of us remained to work on the JCAHO standards–did so, not because we were looking for abuse but because of our belief that sincerity and motivation to improve care is no guarantee of accomplishment. At every NHO conference we held open meetings, and we were under fire for almost every standard. We all held to our belief that standards would maximize the chance that hospices could remain viable and consistent with the original values and goals. The issue, then and now, is not how to have a live and functioning hospice, but how to have one which is true to its purpose.

Over the years, only minor revisions have been made to those original NHO standards. The JCAHO-developed hospice standards were used as the basis for a distinct JCAHO hospice accreditation program. That too has changed; first came the demise of that accreditation program followed by the development of general standards which address the needs of the terminally ill in any health care setting. The hospice industry is again asking the question as to whether there should be a distinct national hospice accreditation program.

The evolution of hospice from a movement to an industry occurred in the early 1980s when the Department of Health and Human Services funded the HCFA Hospice Demonstration Program. We were one of the lucky 26 sites chosen. The purpose of the study was to determine the cost and quality effectiveness of hospice care. Four models of hospice care were examined: community based, home health agency based, hospital based, and freestanding hospices. Five of the 26 were in California.

The essential components of the Medicare Hospice Benefit originated with the Demonstration Project. It was a glorious time: patients and families received unlimited services, sometimes to an embarrassing extent. There were virtually no limitations on care. Before the completion of the Hospice Demonstration Project, Don Gaetz and Hugh Westbrook, whose Hospice Inc. in Miami was a site, began an organizing campaign to pass federal legislation creating this new benefit for Medicare beneficiaries.

This became one of the most contentious periods in the life of the National Hospice Organization. It was obvious to many that reimbursement for service was crucial to the survival and growth of this fledgling movement. The means to that end were the source of the controversy. My naivete about the road to legislative success was a reason I called so loudly for an open process as one set of hospice leaders began crafting this new benefit. Nevertheless, a tremendous amount of time and energy was spent fighting for the chance to be heard. The outcome was not only reimbursement for hospice care, but also ultimately, the "legitimization" of hospice care in the medical system. As hospice care was integrated into the health care system, by virtue of its reimbursement, the medical community finally began to accept hospice.

Another outcome of federal reimbursement was the dilemma confronting many community based hospice programs: whether or not to seek Medicare certification and accept payment for their services. There was grave concern that money, to say nothing of the accompanying regulations governing the acceptance of that money, would forever alter the hospice program. Programs also resisted this change because of the inevitable reporting, accountability and regulations imposed as conditions of federal dollars. Many programs initially chose to continue to rely on community support to fund their program.

Hospices were slow to seek Medicare certification and HCFA and Congress expressed concern and surprise at the slow pace with which programs were becoming certified. Many new entrant providers from more traditional healthcare institutions began to see the potential for a financially viable program and as hospice programs began to proliferate, Medicare certification became a necessity in order to offer comparable benefits.

HOSPICE WITHIN HOME HEALTH AGENCY

My experience developing a hospice program within a large home health agency was somewhat different from those who were creating a community based hospice program. It was clear to me from the beginning that if our hospice program was going to succeed, we had to become an integral part of the existing system. Hospital Home Health Care Agency was a cooperative effort of 10 hospitals and if we criticized the aggressive approach that many community hospitals had towards terminally ill patients, we couldn't expect any referrals or cooperation from those hospitals. Whereas many early hospice providers were sharply critical of hospital care for dying patients, our approach was decidedly low key.

Most of our registered nurses and social workers, home health aides, and psychologist were paid employees; our medical director, pharmacists, chaplain, and volunteer director were initially volunteers. When a patient met the home health criteria, we could bill for covered services, thus generating some revenue for the program. With financial support pieced together from grants and the home health agency, meeting payroll was not the constant worry faced by many other hospice administrators.

My challenge in the home health agency included defining and defending hospice as distinct from traditional home care. To this day, I believe that the preferred model is a team of nurses and social workers who care exclusively for terminally ill patients. Those who choose this work, as opposed to being assigned to care for dying patients, bring a passion and commitment which sustains them in this demanding job. Working as an interdisciplinary team also requires effort on everyone's part. Certainly, team members express that it often seems easier to do the job "myself"; however, the contribution of other perspectives, skills and disciplines is critical to the success of hospice. I tell every employee that no one can do this work alone. Your team members are who you must rely on and turn to. Those staff who cannot embrace this model are the ones who "burn out," for the burden of these needy patients and families is simply too much for one person.

I spent considerable time and energy differentiating between hospice and home health. It was recognized that hospice productivity standards must be lower than for home health, the hospice team met every week and support groups for hospice staff are an integral aspect of effective personal and team practice. This differentiation of hospice from home health, coupled with the media coverage highlighting this "special" work, and glowing letters and donations from families created some resentment by home health staff. Hospice staff were viewed as elitist and frequently referred to as "prima donnas." Every hospice relied on community support for survival; those dollars also made it possible to provide essentials and extras for patients and families.

The people who came to work in hospice 23 years ago had the same motivations that staff articulate today. Often there was a close friend and/or family member who died well, with the support and expertise which made it a positive experience, or conversely died a horrible death which was the impetus to "make it better" for someone else. Others are drawn to the work and describe hospice as "the kind of meaningful nursing I have been looking for." They have a passion for caring and are comfortable and willing to apply their skills to assure dying patients the optimal quality of life.

BACK TO THE FUTURE

The public seems even more afraid of death in 1998 than in 1975. As Jeanne Dennis, my colleague and friend for 20 years recently said "hospice is old news . . . and bad news." To a much greater extent today the public knows what hospice is–and increasingly they view it as bad news about their illness and thus a service to be saved for the last few days of life. The recent experience of hospice providers across the country has been that because hospice enters the lives of these patients so late in their illness, we are operating in a crisis mode. We mobilize all resources and focus on the most pressing problems, which are usually pain and symptom management. The emotional and spiritual issues, which usually take longer to address and resolve, often never surface, given the urgency of other concerns. Is that our role? Is that what terminally ill patients need and want? Or do we have a role to play at some earlier point in the patient's illness? The leaders in hospice today need the same energy and commitment to go back where we started–to explore anew the unmet needs of terminally ill patients and their families within the context of health care today.

Today, hospice operates in a health care environment and climate which is rife with suspicion; increasing Medicare expenditures for a growing number of beneficiaries is viewed with alarm by legislators, policymakers and government regulators. After more than a decade of benign neglect, our integration into the health care system has also created an industry that is scrutinized, licensed, accredited, and regulated beyond our wildest dreams. Many of the hospice leaders that I have known for many years can not believe the suspicion that has crept into an industry that was founded on principles of respect, dignity and tolerance. Although patient and family satisfaction with hospice care is remarkably high, given the dissatisfaction most health care consumers express, our reputation has been tarnished in recent years by media reports which have targeted localized abuses and regulatory interpretations which defy logic.

In essence, we are now stepping back to reaffirm our commitment to improve care of the dying. The definition of hospice has expanded beyond the cancer diagnosis to include anyone with a terminal illness and a prognosis of six months or less. This has created nationwide access to hospice care, substantial growth in expenditures for hospice and a governmental focus on tightening the definition of "terminally ill." Many hospice providers believe that retrenchment and limiting access to hospice care is part of the federal agenda. Suddenly, special "fraud alerts" have been issued for hospice and the media has done its best to use a broad brush to put the industry on the defensive.

When the Medicare Hospice Benefit was being created, there was great concern that the accompanying regulations would come to define hospice care in America. To a large extent, that has become true. What is also true is that the changes in the practice of medicine have dramatically impacted the delivery of hospice care since 1983 while the Medicare Hospice Benefit has remained essentially the same.

As a member of the NHO Medicare Benefit and End of Life Committee, I spent the last year with other hospice leaders examining and dissecting the Medicare Hospice Benefit. We listened to hospice providers and other health care providers talk about what is needed now, in this day and age, to care for the terminally ill. We are back at the beginning–trying to improve care at the end of life with a system which is too restrictive. We need to continue our exploring and look beyond the generally accepted definition of hospice and consider where hospice fits in the "end-of-life" discussions currently being held.

One of the most significant changes over the last 20 years is the extent to which there is widespread discussion about, and acknowledgement that care at the end-of-life is still inadequate. Hospice programs cared for 500,000 dying patients in 1997, which is but a small percentage of those eligible. Palliative care medicine is increasingly recognized as a specialty focused on relieving the symptoms of a life threatening illness. The American Medical Association, the Institute of Medicine, and the Robert Wood Johnson Foundation have all developed end-of-life initiatives.

Hospice leaders are in a strong position to participate actively in these forums, for our 20 years of experience in caring for dying patients, give us credibility. We must, however, face the challenge of change. We must review and renew ourselves, for our patients, our society, our health care system, and even the values and beliefs about end of life, have changed. Although we have impacted the life and death of hundreds of thousands of people, our work to improve that care will never be done. In the words of T.S. Eliot:

> *We shall not cease from explorations*
> *And the end to all our exploring*
> *Will be to arrive where we started*
> *And know the place for the first time.*

Reflections on the History of Occupational Stress in Hospice/Palliative Care

Mary L. S. Vachon

SUMMARY. The concept of hospice and palliative care emerged a quarter of a century ago out of recognition of the unmet needs of dying persons and the social issues of the 1960s and 1970s. The issues of the day included the sexual revolution; a questioning of social values; an increased awareness of death resulting from the murder of the Kennedy brothers and Martin Luther King and daily television exposure to deaths in the Vietnam War, feminism, consumerism, reclaiming a more humanized role in the birth process, and hence in the process of death. The history of the hospice movement and the stress experienced by staff is traced from the early developmental days through to the present. Initially there was sometimes a struggle to integrate the concepts of relief of physical symptoms with meeting the psychosocial and emotional needs of patients and families, caregivers were expected to sacrifice much of their personal life for work, emotional intensity was high and supports were developed to ease some of the stress experienced by caregivers. From the early days team stress and burnout have been issues of concern. In the 1980s issues involved establishing funding sources, dealing with the new crisis of AIDS, and dealing with the gap between the ideal and the real. In the 1990s the economic climate has escalated some of the tensions that have always existed as hospice attempts to position itself within mainstream care with diminishing fiscal resources. These are issues that confront us as we move into the next century. *[Article copies available for a fee from The Haworth Document Delivery Service: 1-800-342-9678. E-mail address: getinfo@haworthpressinc. com <Website: http://www.haworthpressinc.com>]*

[Haworth co-indexing entry note]: "Reflections on the History of Occupational Stress in Hospice/Palliative Care." Vachon, Mary L. S. Co-published simultaneously in *The Hospice Journal* (The Haworth Press, Inc.) Vol. 14, No. 3/4, 1999, pp. 229-246; and: *The Hospice Heritage: Celebrating Our Future* (ed: Inge B. Corless and Zelda Foster) The Haworth Press, Inc., 1999, pp. 229-246. Single or multiple copies of this article are available for a fee from The Haworth Document Delivery Service [1-800-342-9678, 9:00 a.m. - 5:00 p.m. (EST). E-mail address: getinfo@haworthpressinc.com].

KEYWORDS. Hospice, palliative care, occupational stress, burnout

INTRODUCTION

The modern hospice movement in Europe can be seen as dating back to the development of St. Christopher's Hospice in 1967. In North America the movement began in 1974 in the USA, with the opening of the Connecticut Hospice (initially a home care program) and the St. Luke's Hospital consulting team and in Canada with the St. Boniface Terminal Care Unit in Winnipeg, Manitoba and the Royal Victoria Hospital Palliative Care Unit in Montreal, Quebec (Saunders, 1993; Twycross, 1980; Vachon, 1995). This article will present personal reflections on issues related to the social context of the development of hospice and issues related to caregivers and staff stress within this burgeoning social phenomenon over the years of my involvement with the movement. More theoretical reviews of the subject can be found elsewhere (Vachon, 1995, 1997, 1998a, b, c). Prior to the emergence of the hospice movement in North America there was a small literature on the care of the dying written by such pioneers as Feifel (1959), Folta (1965), Fox (1959), Glaser and Strauss (1964, 1965, 1968), Hinton (1967), Quint (1966, 1967), Saunders (1959) and Sudnow (1967). Kubler-Ross's landmark book *On Death and Dying* (1969) had appeared and across North America patients were being expected to go through the five prescribed stages of death and dying.

In the early 1970s the field of medical oncology was fairly new. Adjuvant chemotherapy, begun in the 1950s, first proved useful in 1965 (Zubrod, 1979 in Yarbro, 1996). In 1964, the American Society of Clinical Oncology was established to create a forum for the new specialty of medical oncology and nurses became recognized as having an important role in the care of the person with cancer and a key role in the evolving concept of the cancer care team (Yarbro, 1996). Some interventions had begun to help staff care for the dying persons with whom they were working (Artiss & Levine, 1973, Klagsbrun, 1970).

Caregivers of many disciplines involved in the care of the dying and bereaved had begun to meet and present research findings through organizations such as the Foundation of Thanatology at Columbia University under the leadership of Dr. Austin Kutscher. In 1974, Dr. John Fryer and Ken Spillman of the Philadelphia Ars Moriendi group organized the first meeting of what later became the International Work Group on Death, Dying and Bereavement. This meeting was attended by leaders in the field from around the world. Dr. Cecily Saunders spoke about St. Christopher's Hospice, Florence Wald shared issues involving the development of the Connecticut Hospice and Dr. Balfour Mount spoke of the development of the Palliative Care Unit at the Royal Victoria Hospital. Dr. Robert Jay Lifton presented his work on *Home from the War,* an analysis of veterans who returned from the Vietnam War (Lifton, 1973). The conceptual model of his book is of death and the continuity of life-a model that also underpinned hospice.

THE CULTURE OF THE TIMES

The sexual revolution had begun in the 1960s; homosexuality and heterosexuality were more openly discussed than they had been in previous generations. AIDS was an unknown phenomenon. The values of society were being seriously questioned, especially by its younger members. These were the days of hippies, free love, drugs, Kent State, the murders of John and Robert Kennedy, and Martin Luther King, the Vietnam War, the message not to trust bureaucracy and anyone over 30. Man had gone to the moon. There was the sense that the sky was the limit, money was, or should be, available to do what needed to be done. People just needed to love one another. If you wanted something done–then just go and do it. The times "they were a-changing."

There was a certain arrogance about having conquered many of the diseases known to society. Arnold Toynbee was quoted as saying that death was "un-American" (Stoddard, 1978). It was said that people did not die, they "got deaded"–someone had goofed, death should not happen. Technology reigned, death was going to be overcome. Those who died were isolated in rooms at the end of the corridor. It was commonly stated that sex had come out of the closet, now it was time for death to come out of the closet. It was time to talk about death, to acknowledge that people did die and to improve the care of the dying.

The early days of openly dealing with death and dying were intense. Sex and death were intertwined. One of the questions being asked, and not answered, at an early meeting of leading experts in the field of thanatology was whether or not one slept with one's dying patients. A young therapist reflected that he was working with a dying adolescent girl who was upset that not only was she dying, but she was still a virgin. He felt torn about whether he should try to meet her sexual needs. Another participant was providing sexual surrogates for dying older people.

In the early 1970s the Vietnam War was drawing to a close. Some of the younger people who became involved in the early days of hospice had been involved in dodging the draft, others had been conscientious objectors, or had been in the war and were forever touched by it. Many were challenging the traditional beliefs of society. With the Vietnam War and nearly universal access to television in the United States and Canada, for the first time death had come into homes as a nightly occurrence on the 6:00 news. There was a desire to make death more meaningful than death in Vietnam and death in highly technological hospitals seemed to be.

In addition, consumers had become more active in the 1960s and early 1970s. The self help movement was flourishing. The Women's Movement was in full swing. Nurses were expanding their roles and attempting to become more collaborative partners in care with physicians (Vachon, Lyall, Rogers, 1976). Women were becoming more assertive and pushing to change the assumptions under which they had been leading their lives. They were assuming an active role in childbirth and fighting to have partners present for deliveries. Births were sometimes taking place at home. As we were reclaiming a role in the natural process of birth, many also wanted to assume a more active role in the universal experience of death. As birth could occur at home or in more humane health care settings, so too might death occur at home, or in more home-like settings, such as hospices.

PERSONAL INVOLVEMENT IN HOSPICE CARE

Early childhood experiences led to my initial interest in death and grief. My nursing school days at Massachusetts General Hospital made me aware of the work of Drs. Erich Lindemann on bereavement (1944), and Avery Weisman and Thomas Hackett on predilection to death (1961). In 1969 I had immigrated to Canada with my husband as draft dodgers. In 1971, I was working at the Clarke Institute of Psychiatry in Toronto when a question to my department head, Dr. Stanley J.J. Freeman, about being helpful to a friend who was soon to die leaving a young family, led to my becoming involved in Princess Margaret Hospital with my colleague, Dr. Alan Lyall.

We were invited to investigate the stress of staff working with cancer patients and to develop programs of intervention for staff members (Rochester, Vachon, Lyall, 1974; Vachon, 1976; Vachon, Lyall, Freeman, 1978). This work led to additional studies of intervention with cancer patients, women with breast cancer and newly widowed women (Vachon and Lyall, 1976; Vachon, Lyall, Rogers et al., 1980; Vachon, Lyall, Rogers et al., 1981-1982).

My introduction to the hospice/palliative care movement began one day in 1974 when Dr. Lyall returned from a medical meeting saying that he had met a young urologist, Dr. Balfour Mount, who had a vision of opening a unit at the Royal Victoria Hospital in Montreal, Quebec to care for the terminally ill. The unit was to be based in part on a model developed in London by Dr. Cecily Saunders at St. Christopher's Hospice. Quebec is primarily a French speaking province. The word "hospice" translated as "poor house" in French so Dr. Mount looked for a new term and developed the concept of a "palliative care" unit. To palliate is to "alleviate (disease) without curing" (Health and Welfare Canada, 1981, p. 1). Dr. Lyall suggested to Dr. Mount that since our team had already studied the stress of staff at Princess Margaret Hospital we might study the stress of the staff of the newly developing Royal Victoria Hospital palliative care unit.

THE 1970s–
DEVELOPMENTAL ISSUES
IN THE EARLY DAYS

Dr. Saunders identified the crucial components of hospice care before St. Christopher's was developed. These were:

- Educating and training medical, nursing, and allied health personnel to be sensitive to the rights, needs, and problems of patients with terminal illnesses;
- Discovering new therapies for managing pain and other discomforts of the terminally ill;
- Providing home care so patients can remain at home as long as they desire and be able to die there if they wish and it is feasible; and

- Attending to both the immediate and the long-term needs of grieving survivors (Saunders, 1959 in Butler, 1979).

As hospice and palliative care programs developed in North America, they struggled to find their own way. In the United States where the movement progressed faster than in Canada, professionals and volunteers worked hand in hand planning to develop programs specific for their community. Stoddard observed "(t)he movement is one, essentially of professional people in the health-care fields who find the present situation intolerable, who discover support for their view among members of the clergy and enlightened laypeople, and who are willing to devote enormous amounts of time, energy, and personal sacrifice to the cause of providing better and more appropriate care in the future, to the terminally ill" (Stoddard, 1978, p. 174).

The hospice movement was said to "focus long overdue attention on how individuals and society as a whole deal with dying and death." Hospice was to be "an embodiment of the finest of human qualities–affection, decency, and kindness . . . less an acceptance of death than an affirmation of a full, complete life" (Butler, 1979, p. 2). By 1977 there were about 70 hospices that were either developed or in process of developing in the United States. Twenty-two of these teams were in California. Most were founded by nurses and physicians planning to offer skilled home care to the terminally ill, hoping over time to develop inpatient units (Stoddard, 1978).

In Canada hospice developed more slowly, in part because of issues related to funding. There were a few volunteer programs, some units in general hospitals, and the occasional free standing hospice. In 1979, National Health and Welfare, Canada formed a subgroup on palliative care services to develop guidelines and recommendations concerning the nature, scope and character of palliative care services (Ajemian and Mount, 1980).

In the early days, physicians, nurses and other health care professionals either did all of their work as volunteers, trying to get hospices up and running, or were paid a small salary and volunteered many hours more than those for which they were paid. Voluntary programs sometimes provided direct service and other times focused on stimulating other voluntary and service organizations to provide expanded coverage; generating financial support for individuals or existing institutions; organizing telephone support networks, or fostering volunteer training. The main disadvantage was that volunteer programs generally could not function adequately for meeting the spectrum of needs faced by the terminally ill and their families (Davidson, 1985).

Hospice programs, operating on no money or minimal funds, often expected major sacrifices and long unpaid volunteer hours serving clients. The work itself was to be the reward. We debated about the impact this work would have on the young children many of us were raising. What would it be like to be raised in a family where death was a common topic of conversation or where a parent was frequently absent because a dying patient was felt to have a greater immediate need than the day-to-day concerns of children or other family members? I remember one young nurse speaking of how drained she felt returning home at the end of a day of dealing with dying hospice clients to confront her husband and two young children. She repeatedly gave them the message that they must nurture her in order for her to be able to go back and nurture her clients the next day. Eventually her family tired of this role and asked her why she kept coming home if she had nothing to give. She decided that her dying patients needed her more than her healthy family, left her family to minister to her clients and soon left hospice work, finding that she had nothing left to give to anyone.

People who went on to become leaders in the field, spoke of not taking a salary for several years, mortgaging homes to cover financial responsibilities, sacrificing marriages and finally reaching the stage of realizing that there had to be some realistic limits set on their work and that professionals would need to be paid living wages if they were going to continue to function in the field.

The first and second generation hospice caregivers were a dedicated and intense group. The early meetings were often emotional and cathartic. People would see one another at meetings, hug and burst into tears, carrying considerable unresolved grief for all the people they had cared for who had died. The initial meetings were sometimes high on emotional issues and somewhat short on scientific theory. There was sometimes a struggle to combine psychosocial, spiritual issues with good relief of physical symptoms. Many volunteer programs had minimal or no connection with professionals. They did what they could with the resources they had and struggled with the best ways to provide care.

As the movement progressed, there was some tension as meetings became more "scientific and professional" and some participants wondered if hospice was losing its heart. Meanwhile hospices were experiencing significant growing pains. New hospices sprung up rapidly in some communities without sufficient groundwork having been done to assess the need for the program. Dr. Mount was quoted as referring to the "Kentucky Fried Hospice Movement," the idea of a hospice on every block. Often the people who had the charisma and creativity to develop a hospice did not have the knowledge and skills to carry their ideas into day-to-day practice. It was not unusual for those who founded hospices to return from a vacation to find they had been "ousted" by the Board of Directors.

While people talked about openness, often the expression of anger and conflict was suppressed and emerged in painful ways. In one meeting staff spoke of the way their hospice director would handle anger–by hugging everyone in the staff meeting, except the person she was angry with. "Hospice hugging" was an issue in the early days. Hugging was just beginning to become more socially acceptable. Caregivers would go to another person saying that the other person "needed a hug," this was sometimes interpreted as someone else deciding what you needed when you did not yourself feel that this was what you needed. Feelings of anger could be experienced and if the person withdrew from the hug, she was perceived as being the person with the problem, as opposed to the "hugger" overstepping boundaries.

In the early days there were struggles with hospice staff and volunteers feeling that they "knew" how things should be done and how people "should" die. Underneath all the loving was sometimes a strong need for control. When reality did not meet a caregiver's expectations–when patients did not want to make peace before they died, or wanted to continue active treatment when caregivers felt they should accept the reality of impending death–there was sometimes difficulty. This conflict was the source of some of the tension that emerged when patients began to come home to die or transfer into a hospice unit, while still wanting to receive such treatments as IVs, TPN, or chemotherapy. These were the days when the primary issue was what patients should "want" to have as opposed to having limited resources and needing to fit into the regulations of managed care.

In the early stages, the hospice movement experienced opposition from powerful political forces initially from medicine and nursing and later from the for-profit, health care corporations. The National Hospice Organization was formally established in 1979 to promote the hospice concept in the United States and to set standards for hospice care.

THE EARLY DAYS-THE RESEARCH

In 1974 our team began to study the stress of the staff of the Royal Victoria Hospital Palliative Care Unit (PCU). My colleagues, Dr. Alan Lyall, Joy Rogers and I visited the staff before the unit opened and at two to three month intervals over the first 15 months of the service's development. The stress of the PCU staff was compared with that of other staff at the Royal Victoria Hospital as well as with widows, and women with breast cancer.

Three months after the development of the palliative care unit, the nursing staff had scores on the Goldberg General Health Questionnaire (GHQ) (Goldberg, 1978) that were twice as high as those of the nurses on the other units and about half the score of women newly diagnosed with breast cancer. The scores of the palliative care staff were very similar to those of newly widowed women (9.4 vs. 10) (Lyall, Rogers, Vachon, 1976; Lyall, Vachon, Rogers, 1980). Over the following ten months the stress decreased to negligible levels. Analysis of the data showed that those who were most stressed left the PCU. Those who stayed had lower stress scores from the beginning. Stressors from interpersonal problems among staff and inadequate support from other staff declined over time. Several other areas disappeared entirely: difficulty with the rest of the hospital, a sense of personal inadequacy and not knowing what was expected on the job. Other problems decreased but continued to be areas of concern: facing the death of a patient, difficulty dealing with families, and watching patients suffer. Some of the factors associated with staying or leaving the service included: being more religious, and being more "venturesome" or "spontaneous," as opposed to "shy" on the 16 Personality Factor scale (Cattell, Eber, Tatsuoka, 1970).

In the early days, the reasons professional staff gave for choosing to work with the dying, either in a hospice or oncology, included: having come into the work purely by accident or convenience; a desire to do the "in thing" or to affiliate with a charismatic leader; an intellectual appeal; a desire for mastery over death; a sense of "calling"; previous personal experience; and a suspicion that they might someday develop a similar disease (Vachon, 1979a).

Hospice volunteers were found to have turned to hospice work after experiencing the death of a significant other, to have a positive view of family and friends, to have a professional interest in counseling or a related profession, and to be satisfied or very satisfied with their spiritual lives. They found it helpful to have empathic contact with clients, to turn inward to focus on themselves and their clients, to recognize their good work, receive support from family and friends and to engage in physical activity (Garfield and Jenkins, 1981-2). Other early studies of staff stress found that *inpatient staff* experienced stress from dealing with families, identifying with patients, their relationship with administration and with patients needing to return to the hospital to die. *Home care hospice nurses* had difficulty with monitoring medications and managing respiratory symptoms at home, explaining death to children, dealing with depressed patients and patients with whom they identified, and difficult work and on-call schedules (Barstow, 1980); team conflict, role conflict, role ambiguity and constant exposure to dying (Mount and Voyer, 1980); lack of staff support, emotional concerns for patients and families and management of the disease process (Yancik, 1984).

Issues of role ambiguity were a major problem in the early days as the role of professional and volunteer were not clearly defined. Not only were professionals often working long hours without financial recompense, there were also not clearly established boundaries between the roles of professional and friend with clients. Even today the roles between professionals, volunteers and clients often have more role blurring than is found in other specialties. However, over time there has been somewhat more recognition of the need to set some appropriate boundaries, taking into account the limitations of individuals (Vachon, 1995).

In the largest early study of staff stress 1,281 staff were surveyed for the National Hospice Study (Masterson-Allen, Mor, Laliberte, Monteiro, 1985; Mor and Laliberte, 1984). The burnout rate was low, but was found to be more common in those aged under 40, with a higher level of education, with long tenure and who worked full-time.

Turnipseed (1987) suggested that staff working in hospice might have less burnout because, whereas burnout is the result of "chronic stress of consistent or repeated emotional pressure associated with an intense involvement with people over long periods of time" (Pines & Aronson, 1988), hospice nurses more often reported organizational or staff support stress than stress arising from patients and families.

From the early days of hospice the team was identified as one of the biggest stressors, and the place where stress was often manifest, but teamwork was also found to be one of the major coping mechanisms for hospice staff (Vachon, 1987). A team of idealistic people coming together because of a perceived deficiency in the system and driven to make changes sometimes carried their own unresolved issues. A quote attributed to Dr. Cicely Saunders in the early days of the hospice movement "If you say you work in a hospice team, you have to be willing to show your battle scars" is still true today.

Regular team meetings were found to be important to set goals to accomplish the work of the team, provide a time of evaluation and reflection on the work being accomplished, and allow for shared decision-making (Barstow, 1980, Munley, 1985, Vachon, 1987). Staff support was also seen to be integral to effective palliative care. It was hypothesized, even in the early research that these buffers might serve to mitigate the stress that would otherwise be seen to be more evident (Masterson-Allen, Mor, Laliberte, 1985; Vachon, 1986; Vachon, 1987).

THE 1980s–THE MID YEARS

A few experiences stand out from the mid-years of the movement–discussions about what the implications would be of applying for Medicare funding? What would happen when services were "capped", or when people could be involved in hospice for only a limited period of time? What about for-profit hospices–would they take the heart out of hospice? I gave what was said to be the first lecture ever to nurses from the Japan Nurses' Association on the subject of nurses stress in the care of the terminally ill in 1987. I was in Zimbabwe in 1988 when it was announced that the first case of AIDS had just been discovered in that country. In reality, a busy AIDS clinic had been operating for some time–the problem simply wasn't being acknowledged by those in positions of authority.

In 1979 I was invited to write a book on occupational stress in the care of the dying (Vachon, 1987). The data was gathered from a convenience sample of almost 600 people from around the world. As I traveled to lecture I interviewed people. The data was gathered from 1980-1983, the book was written from 1983-1985. When I reviewed the page proofs in 1986-1987 I was shocked to realize that as I had interviewed all these people the phenomenon of AIDS had been developing. No one I had interviewed had even mentioned the issue that had become a major problem on the world stage by 1987.

Of the total of almost 600 caregivers interviewed, 60 worked in palliative care. The major stressors they identified were: communication problems with "others" in the system, role ambiguity, team communication problems, administrative communication problems and role conflict. The problems with "others" in the system had a lot to do with hospice staff being concerned that patients were not being referred to them at all or they were not being referred early enough. A comment that typified some of the rivalry between hospice and oncology staff came from a hospice caregiver who was angry that oncology staff were coming to the hospice meetings and trying to learn about the concepts of pain management. This was considered to be quite inappropriate, as the concepts of good pain management were felt to belong exclusively to hospice. If oncology staff could learn such concepts they might not refer patients to hospice and the concept would fail. Somehow the needs of the patient got a bit lost in this discussion.

Over 100 hospice workers attending the 1986 national conference entitled "Hospice Management Interdisciplinary Team Development" were asked to identify the motivation and personality characteristics that attracted people to work in palliative care. Their comments reflect the American experience at that time. The participants felt that some of their members were rebels with a great desire to make changes-sometimes these changes were carefully thought out and these so called "rebels" developed innovative programs that did much to meet the needs of patients, families and communities. At other times, however, the proposed programs fell apart because of the development of rival factions, or because of fiscal constraints or the organizational skills of those being attracted to the field not being sufficient for the task of organizational development. Some people were attracted to the field because of a sense of "enlightened opportunism"; it looked as if this was a good place to be at this particular point in time. People achieved local, national and even international, recognition, in part because of an ability to present a need for hospice care.

Some came into hospice care because of a religious commitment.

At the time it was not uncommon to feel that one must have a spiritual base in order to survive in hospice work. Certain types of religious motives were experienced negatively by some team members who saw their colleagues as being "religious zealots"–out to make death bed conversions. Some were labeled by their colleagues as being "intensity vultures," who required the "high" that came from constant association with life and death. Other personality characteristics that were identified included: the need to prove that "I'm OK; the previous problems that I have had within the system were not my fault but the fault of the system, and working in a hospice will allow me to correct all these wrongs." There was also a group who were attracted because of the need to receive nurturing from the system and from their colleagues (Vachon, 1995).

In the 1980s a number of stressors associated with hospice work were identified. These included: the nature of the work with clients and families, including dealing with dying patients and those struggling to accept death (Gotay et al., 1985; Munley, 1985 Krikorian and Moser, 1985; Paradis et al., 1987; Power and Sharp, 1988; Paradis and Usui, 1989); the struggle to narrow the gap between "real" and "ideal" and frustrations with the attempt to provide quality care (Munley, 1985; Krikorian and Moser, 1985; Power and Sharp, 1988; Paradis and Usui, 1989); problems with symptom relief (Gotay et al., 1985); feelings of personal inadequacy (Paradis et al., 1987); insufficient information and preparation (Paradis et al., 1987; Power and Sharp, 1988; Paradis and Usui, 1989); giving effective psychosocial support (Gotay et al., 1985; Power and Sharp, 1988); environmental and bureaucratic issues (Munley, 1985; Krikorian and Moser, 1985); role strain (Munley, 1985); team conflict (Paradis and Usui, 1989); role ambiguity in volunteers (Paradis et al., 1987); feeling a lack of support (Paradis et al., 1987); and difficulty working with volunteers (Paradis and Usui, 1989).

THE 1990s

Communication problems with "others in the system" including other departments, general practitioners and other hospices have been recognized as issues and may become worse with the current economic climate. Internationally, caregivers report problems encountered trying to position their hospice/palliative care programs within the changing health care environment. Rivalries are encountered as programs try to determine with which agencies, if any, they will have preferred partner arrangements. The aggressive marketing techniques of some hospice programs have resulted in conflicts amongst the programs existing in and/or developing within some communities. This problem is undoubtedly more pronounced in the United States (Vachon, 1998a).

As palliative care became a specialty in the United Kingdom and palliative care physicians began to assume a more active role in directing hospice and palliative care programs conflicts between nurses and physicians have emerged. Hospice medical directors rated their relationships with the matron as being most problematic (Finlay, 1990). In a large study of specialist physicians, including palliative care physicians, "encountering difficulties in relationships with nurses" was the only aspect of work in which palliative care physicians reported more stress than their colleagues in other specialties. This was hypothesized to derive in part from the lack of role clarity in the roles of consultants and senior nurses in palliative care, since historically some charitably-funded hospices were run by matrons (Graham, Ramirez, Cull et al., 1996). Hospice matrons report a lack of participation in decision-making and planning (Alexander and MacLeod, 1992) and a lack of decision-making was implicated in high levels of depression in British hospice nurses (Cooper and Mitchell, 1990). Nursing staff reported difficulty in fulfilling their own performance expectations and felt pressured into a continuous commitment of time and energy to care for the dying because of the belief that the time to care is brief and the process happening *now* is the only meaningful measure of having cared well for this patient (McWilliam, Burdock, Wamsley, 1993).

Role strain was experienced by palliative care physicians, 35% of whom felt insufficiently trained in communication skills and 81% felt insufficiently trained in management skills. Burnout was more prevalent among consultants who felt insufficiently trained in communication and management skills (Graham, Ramirez, Cull et al., 1996). Palliative care physicians report less stress than other consultants from aspects of work involving communicating with patients and relatives in difficult situations and having good relationships with patients, relatives and staff was regarded as their greatest source of job satisfaction (Graham, Ramirez, Cull et al., 1996).

A SUMMARY OF THE LITERATURE

A review of the research literature from the early days of the movement concluded that while high stress was identified as a problem in the early days of the movement, later studies have shown that stress and burnout in palliative care are by no means universal. Staff stress in hospice and palliative care were found to be less than that in many other settings. However, other studies have noted suicidal ideation (Finlay, 1990), increased alcohol and drug usage (Finlay, 1990), anxiety (Cooper and Mitchell, 1990) and depression (Finlay, 1990; Alexander and MacLeod, 1992) and difficulty in dealing with issues of death and dying (Foxall et al., 1990; Bené and Foxall, 1991). It is hypothesized that part of the reason that stress may be lower than expected in some settings was the early recognition of the potential stress inherent in this field and the development of appropriate organizational and personal coping strategies to deal with identified stressors. Staff in hospice/palliative care have been found to have increased stress when mechanisms such as social support, involvement in decision-making, and a realistic workload are not available. The stress in palliative care was found to be due in large measure to organizational and social issues, although personal issues were also found to have an influence (Vachon, 1995).

The major problems in palliative care today are probably more related to issues of reimbursement, the economic issues of society, government and insurance intervention into the determination of who should be offered palliative care and how services and expectations should be determined, conflict and rivalry with other specialties, referral practices, deciding how "active" palliative care should be, team conflict and determining the role of hospice in the current health care environment. While these issues are not totally new to the field, they are assuming increasing importance as we enter into the next century.

REFERENCES

Ajemian, I., Mount, B.M. (1980). Preface. In I. Ajemian and B.M. Mount (eds). *The R.V.H. Manual on Palliative/Hospice Care*. New York: ARNO Press.

Alexander, D.A., MacLeod, M. (1992). Stress among palliative care matrons: a major problem for a minority group. *Palliat Med* 6: 111-124.

Artiss, K.L., Levine, A. (1973). Doctor-patient relationship in severe illness. *N Engl J Med* 288(23): 1210-1214.

Barstowe, J. (1980). Stress variance in hospice nursing. *Nurs Outlook* 28:751-54.

Bené, B., Foxall, M.J. (1991). Death anxiety and job stress in hospice and medical-surgical nurses. *Hosp J* 7(3): 25-41.

Butler, R.N. (1979). The need for quality hospice care. *Qual Rev Bull* 5(5): 2-7.

Cattell, R.B.; Eber, H.W.; Tatsuoka, M.M. (1970). *Handbook for the Sixteen Personality Factor Questionnaire (16PF)*. Champaign, IL: Institute for Personality and Ability Testing.

Cooper C.L., Mitchell S. (1990). Nursing the critically ill and dying. *Hum Relations* 43: 297-311.

Davidson, G.W. (1985). Introduction. In G.W. Davidson (ed). *The Hospice: Development and Administration*, 2nd edition. Washington, D.C.: Hemisphere Publishing Corporation, 1-12.

Feifel, H. (1959). *The Meaning of Death*. New York: Blakiston Division, McGraw-Hill.

Finlay, I.G. (1990). Sources of stress in hospice medical directors and matrons. *Palliat Med* 4:5-9.

Folta, J. R. (1965). The perception of death. *Nurs Res* 14:233-235.

Fox, R.C. (1959). *Experiment Perilous*. Glencoe, IL: The Free Press.

Foxall, M.J.; Zimmerman, L.; Standley, R.; Bené B. (1990). A comparison of frequency and sources of nursing job stress perceived by intensive care, hospice and medical-surgical nurses. *J Adv Nurs* 15: 577-584.

Garfield, C.A., Jenkins, G.J. (1981-2). Stress and coping of volunteers counseling the dying and bereaved. *Omega* 12: 1-13.

Glaser, B.G., Strauss, A.L. (1964). Awareness contexts and social interaction. *Am Soc Rev* 29: 669-679.

Glaser, B.G., Strauss, A.L. (1965). *Awareness of Dying*. Chicago: Aldine.

Glaser, B.G., Strauss, A.L. (1968). *Time for Dying*. Chicago: Aldine.

Goldberg, D. (1978). *Manual of the General Health Questionnaire*. Windsor: NFER-Nelson.

Gotay, C.C.; Crockett, S.; West, C. (1985) Palliative home care nursing: Nurses' perceptions of roles and stress. *Can Ment Health* 33: 6-9.

Graham, J.; Ramirez, A.J.; Cull, A. ; Gregory, W.M.; Finlay, I.; Hoy, A.; Richards, M.A. (1996). Job stress and satisfaction among palliative physicians. *Palliat Med* 10: 185-194.

Health and Welfare Canada (1981). *Report of the Working Group on Special Services in Hospitals*. Ottawa: Health Services Directorate Health Services and Promotion Branch.

Hinton, J. (1967). *Dying*. Baltimore: Penquin.

Klagsbrun, S. (1970). Cancer, emotions and nurses. *Am J Psychiat* 126: 1237-1244.

Krikorian, D.A., Moser, D.H. (1985). Satisfactions and stresses experienced by professional nurses in hospice programs. *Am J Hosp Care* 2(1):25-33.

Kübler-Ross, E.G. (1969). *On Death and Dying*. Toronto: Collier-Macmillan.

Lifton, R.J. (1973). *Home from the War*. New York: Simon and Schuster.

Lindemann, E. (1944). Symptomatology and management of acute grief. *Am J Psychiatry* 101: 141-148.

Lyall, W.A.L.; Rogers J.; Vachon M.L.S. (1976). Report to the Palliative Care Unit of the Royal Victoria Hospital regarding professional stress in the care of the dying. In B.M. Mount (ed). *Palliative Care Service Oct. 1976 Report.* Montreal: Royal Victoria Hospital, 457-68.

Lyall, W.A.L.; Vachon, M.L.S.; Rogers, J. (1980). A study of the degree of stress experienced by professionals caring for dying patients. In I. Ajemian and B. M. Mount (eds). *The R.V.H. Manual on Palliative/Hospice Care.* New York: ARNO Press. 498-507.

Masterson-Allen, S.; Mor, V.; Laliberte, L.; Monteiro, L. (1985). Staff burnout in a hospice setting. *Hosp J* 1: 1-15.

McWilliam, C.L.; Burdock, J.; Wamsley, J. (1993). The challenging experience of palliative care support-team nursing. *Onc Nurs Forum* 20: 770-785.

Mor, V., Laliberte, L. (1984). Burnout among hospice staff. *Health Soc Work* 9: 274-283.

Mount, B.M., Voyer, J. (1980). Staff stress in palliative/hospice care. In I. Ajemian and B. M. Mount (eds). *The RVH Manual on Palliative/Hospice Care.* New York: ARNO Press, 457-488.

Munley, A. (1985). Sources of hospice staff stress and how to cope with it. *Nurs Clin N Am* 20:343-355.

Paradis, L.F.; Miller, B.; Runnion, V.M. (1987). Volunteer stress and burnout: Issues for administrators. *Hosp J* 3:165-183.

Paradis, L.F., Usui, W.M. (1989). Hospice staff and volunteers: Issues for management. *J Psychosoc Oncol* 7:121-139.

Pines. A.M., Aronson, E. (1988*) Career burnout: causes and cures.* New York: Free Press.

Power, K.G., Sharp, G.R. (1988). A comparison of sources of nursing stress and job satisfaction among mental handicap and hospice nursing staff. *J Adv Nurs* 13: 726-732.

Quint, J.C. (1966). Awareness of death and the nurse's composure. *Nurs Res* 15: 49-55.

Quint, J.C. (1967). When patients die: some nursing problems. *Can Nurs* 63(12): 33-36.

Rochester, S.R.; Vachon, M.L.S.; Lyall, W.A.L. (1974). Immediacy in language: a channel to the care of the dying patient. *J Comm Psychol* 2:1: 75-76.

Saunders, C. (1959). *Care of the Dying.* London: Macmillan.

Saunders, C. (1993). Foreword. In D. Doyle, G.W. Hanks, N. MacDonald (eds). *Oxford Textbook of Palliative Medicine.* Oxford: Oxford University Press, v-viii.

Stoddard, S. (1978). The Hospice Maverenl. Briarcliff Manor, NY: Stein & Day.

Sudnow, D. (1967). Passing On: *The Social Organization of Dying.* Englewood Cliffs, N.J.: Prentice-Hall.

Turnipseed, D.L. (1987). Burnout among hospice nurses: an empirical assessment. *Hosp J* 3(2/3): 105-119.

Twycross, R.G. (1980). Hospice care–redressing the balance in medicine. *J R Soc Med* 73: 475-81.

Vachon, M.L.S. (1976). Enforced proximity to stress in the client environment. *Can Nurs* 72: 40 43.

Vachon M.L.S.; Lyall W.A.L.; Rogers J. (1976). The nurse in thanatology: What she can learn from the women's liberation movement. In A. Earle, N.T. Argondizzo, A.H. Kutscher (eds). *The Nurse as Caregiver for the Dying Patient and His Family.* New York: Columbia University Press, 175-194.

Vachon, M.L.S., Lyall, W.A.L. (1976). Applying Psychiatric Techniques to Patients with Cancer. *Hosp Comm Psych* 27:582-584.

Vachon, M.L.S.; Lyall, W.A.L.; Freeman, S.J.J. (1978). Measurement and management of stress in health professionals working with advanced cancer patients. *Death Ed* 1:365-375.

Vachon, M.L.S. (1979a). Motivation and stress experienced by staff working with the terminally ill. *Death Ed* 2: 113-122.

Vachon, M.L.S. (1979b). Staff Stress in the Care of the Terminally Ill. *Qual Rev Bull* 5: 13-17.

Vachon, M.L.S.; Lyall, W.A.L.; Rogers, J.; Freedman, K.; Freeman, S.J.J. (1980). A controlled study of self-help intervention for widows. *Am J Psychiatr* 137: 1380-1384.

Vachon, M.L.S.; Lyall, W.A.L.; Rogers, J.; Cochrane, J.; Freeman, S.J.J. The Effectiveness of Psychosocial Support During Post-Surgical Treatment of Breast Cancer.(1981-1982). *Int J Psychiat Med* 11: 365-372.

Vachon, M.L.S. (1986). Myths and Realities in Palliative Care. *Hosp J* 2: 63-79.

Vachon, M.L.S. (1987). *Occupational Stress in the Care of the Critically Ill, the Dying and the Bereaved.* New York: Hemisphere.

Vachon, M.L.S. (1995). Staff stress in hospice/palliative care: a review. *Palliat Med* 9: 91-122.

Vachon, M.L.S. (1997). Recent research into staff stress in palliative care. *Eur J Pall Care* 4(3): 99-103.

Vachon, M.L.S. (1998a). The stress of professional caregivers. In D. Doyle, G. Hanks, and N. MacDonald (eds). *Oxford Textbook of Palliative Medicine, 2nd edition.* Oxford: Oxford University Press, 919-929.

Vachon, M.L.S. (1998b). Staff Burnout: Diagnosis, Management and Prevention. In E. Bruera and R.K. Portenoy (eds). *Topics in Palliative Care, Volume 2.* New York: Oxford University Press, 247-293.

Vachon M.L.S. (1998c). Caring for the caregiver in palliative care and oncology. *Sem Onc Nurs.* 14:(2):152-157.

Weisman, A., Hackett, T. (1961). Predelection to death. *Psychosom Med* 23: 232-256.

Yancik, R. (1984). Sources of work stress for hospice staff. *J Psychosoc Oncol* 2(1):21-31.

Yarbro, C.H. (1996). The history of cancer nursing. In R. McCorkle, M. Grant, M. Frank-Stromborg, S.B. Baird (eds). *Cancer Nursing, 2nd edition.* Philadelphia: W.B. Saunders Company, 12-24.

Zubrod, C.G. (1979). Milestones in curative chemotherapy. *Sem Onc* 6: 490-505.

Hospice Reminiscences and Reflections–
An 18 Year Personal
and Professional Love Affair

Ann MacGregor

The foundation of my commitment to the hospice movement recently came into sharp focus. Prior to moving to Mason City, Iowa in January 1967, I served with Project HOPE (Health Opportunity for People Everywhere) for 7 years. Project HOPE began as the dream of William B. Walsh, M.D. He believed that modern American health care education and technology should be shared with the world's developing nations. A hospital ship, which served during the Korean conflict, became the base for the realization of his dream.

The S.S. Hope's first voyage led to my involvement with the project in various nursing and administrative positions, including Chief of Nursing Services. During those years I had the global experience of working in Indonesia, Vietnam, Peru, Ecuador, Guinea West Africa and Nicaragua.

These international health experiences forever changed my views of the human situation, global connectedness and our interdependence. The impact of these experiences, on my personal and professional life, continues to this day.

Serving abroad, I lived in and studied first hand, different cultures, patterns and variations in health care. I observed the continuum of care provided by families facing illness, injury and death. The family, worldwide, was the unit of care. Caring began and continued from the

[Haworth co-indexing entry note]: "Hospice Reminiscences and Reflections–An 18 Year Personal and Professional Love Affair." MacGregor, Ann. Co-published simultaneously in *The Hospice Journal* (The Haworth Press, Inc.) Vol. 14, No. 3/4, 1999, pp. 245-251; and: *The Hospice Heritage: Celebrating Our Future* (ed: Inge B. Corless and Zelda Foster) The Haworth Press, Inc., 1999, pp. 245-251. Single or multiple copies of this article are available for a fee from The Haworth Document Delivery Service [1-800-342-9678, 9:00 a.m. - 5:00 p.m. (EST). E-mail address: getinfo@haworthpressinc.com].

247

cradle to the grave. Time and time again, I witnessed this key mark of our humanness. Without knowing the word for it, I was observing hospice in its purest form.

In 1980, while considering returning to the work force outside of the home, I became aware of the "hospice movement," just beginning in the state of Iowa. In 1981, a local group conducted a needs assessment to determine the feasibility of developing this "new" program for providing care to terminally ill patients and their families. A founding board of directors, of which I was a member, was formed. The rest, as they say, is history. I was fortunate to be in the right place at the right time.

Eighteen years later, as I reflect and reminisce, I feel an overwhelming rush of recall and emotion. My personal and professional life has been enriched beyond description. The beginnings of hospice in north central Iowa mirrors hundreds of similar beginnings in our country. From metropolitan areas to small, rural communities, caring individuals began to talk about how they could improve care of the dying. This dialogue forever changed the pattern of care for terminally ill patients and their families, within the system of health care delivery in the United States.

Conversations took place in living rooms, church basements, hospital committee meetings, the corner coffee shop and many other locations. Recorded minutes of early meetings reveal the fervor, that once released, would know no bounds. Professionals and lay persons came together on common ground, with a central mission and vision. Information about this new "movement" was often stored in a box in someone's car or the corner of a den at home. Office space in those early years was, more often than not, provided gratis by churches and local businesses.

Early funding to sustain such projects was minimal or non-existent. It was not unusual for individuals to be "hired" for specific jobs within the organization without pay. In our program, we had the audacity to advertise in our local newspaper for an initial cadre of employees, with full knowledge that we had no means to provide a paycheck! Even so, we had multiple applications for 2 positions and those first employees worked for several months without reimbursement. In later months, when we issued paychecks, it was not at all unusual for me to question whether I should cash mine or not!

The evolution of the hospice movement over the years was deliberate, focused, halting and uncertain, but sustained. It could not be stopped. Critical to the success of such programs was the networking that provided support and mentoring as we navigated uncharted and often turbulent waters. The foundation which created the structure of such networking, led to the development of state hospice organizations and the National Hospice Organization. Hospice of North Iowa, and hundreds of other programs across the country, owe individual and collective successes in large part, to such organizations. In those early years especially, we learned from each other and shared our successes as well as our failures. Networking among hospices continues but not at the intensity which characterized the early 1980s.

Reflecting and reminiscing on some personal "hospice highlights" includes:

- A meeting in a church basement in Washington, DC, to learn about the basics of the proposed Hospice Medicare Benefit, created a sense of fear, anxiety and uncertainty in those of us attending.
- After achieving Medicare certification and attending the 1984 National Hospice Organization meeting in Hartford, Connecticut, I came away with the distinct sense that the "movement" was on a shaky foundation. I was buoyed however, by the commitment of the "founding zealots" to strengthen the underpinnings and forge ahead.
- In 1986, the First Annual National Hospice Organization Senior Management and Leadership Conference was held in St. Paul, Minnesota. There were approximately 200 in attendance. We felt like one big family. We all knew each other by name. Jay Mahoney was one of a handful of men in attendance, as compared to attendees now.
- Election to the National Hospice Organization Board of Directors as the Northwest Central regional representative and serving for 6 years, was a distinct honor. Serving as chairperson of the board for 2 years during my board tenure provided challenging rewards.
- Two visits to the White House included a special reception given by the First Lady Barbara Bush, in January 1991, in recognition of the important contributions of hospice and a briefing by Presi-

dent Bill Clinton on health care reform in April, 1994. These were special and meaningful events.
- Traveling to London in October 1992, with National Hospice Organization representatives, to present Dame Cicely Saunders the Founders' Award during the celebration of the 25th anniversary of St. Christopher's Hospice, was indeed a highlight.

The complexity of leading a hospice organization in the early eighties pales in comparison to challenges facing hospice leaders in the nineties. The change in the delivery of health care in the United States during the last few years has been ceaseless and chaotic. Transition has been characterized by consolidation, mergers and acquisitions, all seeking in the name of integration, a "seamless continuum of care." For a brief time, some hospice leaders believed our program of care would not succumb to the chaos. The opposite has proven to be true.

Idealism, that characterized early hospice founders and leaders, is being tested by increased regulatory compliance and heightened governmental scrutiny. Financial constraints, the result of numerous external forces, appear to be beyond our control. Some argue that the "heart" of hospice is gone. Some yearn for "the good old days." Others believe that hospice is beginning to look and act like any other "specialty" in the field of health care. Many feel threatened by other organizations that are working to improve end-of-life care for all Americans.

How does a hospice leader, operating in the current environment, maintain the spirit of idealism upon which our foundation was built? Will commitment to that spirit motivate future hospice leaders? As we pass the torch, how will these ideals be maintained and strengthened? Perhaps a review of the next twenty years of hospice history and experience will reveal the answers.

Reflecting on my 18 years in hospice, what I immediately recall are the faces of individuals and stories that I have heard. The commitment and dedication of staff and volunteers is no less today than what it was in the early days of the movement. Patients and families remain our best teachers, and here at the Hospice of North Iowa Center, I see the fulfillment of the hospice mission daily. I observe the people who turn to hospice . . . from every walk of life, age and background. I see babies held by grandparents and dads playing ball on the front lawn with their kids. I see people laughing, struggling, crying, sharing and giving to each other. These are folks like us . . . our neighbors, friends, children, parents and co-workers. Each has something in common–they, or someone they love, is dying. Their needs are multiple and complex. Hospice offers them a haven of comfort and a network of support.

Recalling what I observe and hear, each and every day, I am refreshed and renewed by the courage around me. The quiet heroism of our fellow humans is revealed countless times daily across our country, in the name of hospice.

During my opportunities over the years, to meet with hospice staff and volunteers from across the United States, I have observed common golden threads of excellence that serve as warp and woof in weaving a fabric characterized by distinction and strength. These common threads on the loom of hospice create a beautiful tapestry stretching across broad geographic areas and bridging physical barriers. All of us, in our wonderful diversity, share pride in what has been woven by our work.

As the millennium approaches, I challenge hospice leaders to continue their striving for excellence in the care and caring they give to dying patients and their families. Caring for humans, at the most vulnerable time in their lives, is indeed a sacred trust.

The Moment of Death:
Is Hospice Making a Difference?

Robert Kastenbaum

SUMMARY. The moment of death was a compelling image and dominant concept through much of history. In recent years this term has become destabilized by technological advances and changes in clinical
practice. Perhaps even more significantly, the meanings previously associated with the deathbed scene and the final breath have become increasingly marginalized. Hospice programs continue to demonstrate
that enlightened and dedicated care can markedly reduce the suffering
of terminally ill people and their families. The vast experience acquired
by hospice programs, however, has not yet been translated into a vision
of the moment of death and the deathbed scene for our times. Several
reasons are identified for the limited interest and even more limited
hospice-based research into the deathbed scene and the moment of
death. Hospice programs could contribute much to our understanding
of the final moments of life if this should ever become a priority.
*[Article copies available for a fee from The Haworth Document Delivery Ser-
vice: 1-800-342-9678. E-mail address: getinfo@haworthpressinc.com <Website:
http://www.haworthpressinc.com>]*

KEYWORDS. Ars moriendi, caregivers for the terminally ill, clear
light of death, constructions of dying and death, deathbed scene, hospice-based research, moment of death, observer effect, reluctance to
know, source credibility

*Pages of the calendar slipping away like autumn leaves in a brisk
breeze.* This was once a familiar cinematic device to illustrate the

---

[Haworth co-indexing entry note]: "The Moment of Death: Is Hospice Making a Difference?" Kasten-
baum, Robert. Co-published simultaneously in *The Hospice Journal* (The Haworth Press, Inc.) Vol. 14,
No. 3/4, 1999, pp. 253-270; and: *The Hospice Heritage: Celebrating Our Future* (ed: Inge B. Corless and
Zelda Foster) The Haworth Press, Inc., 1999, pp. 253-270. Single or multiple copies of this article are
available for a fee from The Haworth Document Delivery Service [1-800-342-9678, 9:00 a.m. - 5:00 p.m.
(EST). E-mail address: getinfo@haworthpressinc.com].

passage of time. It would not take a great many falling calendar leaves to represent the history of *The Hospice Journal* and modern palliative care movement, thereby suggesting that there is not much to look back upon. The passage of time can also be measured by change, however. From this standpoint, there is indeed much to reflect upon in the two eventful decades that have been encompassed by *The Hospice Journal.*

The origins and continued growth of the hospice movement have been documented elsewhere (e.g., Stannard, 1978; Phipps, 1988; Saunders & Kastenbaum, 1997), and are frequently revisited in the pages of this *Journal.* Here we focus on a phenomenon that might appear both narrow and archaic: the moment of death. It seems narrow because the *moment of death,* by definition, is but a small part of the complex set of events and experiences that occur during the final phase of life. It may also seem archaic because the mystique of a moment of death comes to us from the perspective of a nearly vanished world. Nevertheless, this narrow and perhaps archaic inquiry could be useful in delineating the core human values, fears, and hopes that have become associated with the transition from life to death. Moreover, the future as well as the past of the palliative care movement is inextricably linked with sociocultural forces and symbol systems whose changing constructions of dying and death have the potential to guide or misguide our efforts.

THE MOMENT OF DEATH: REALITY OR FICTION?

It was once taken as self-evident that a life ends at a clearly perceptible moment, much as a clock strikes the hour. The ancient pedigree of this belief has been renewed frequently by subsequent generations. Death educators, for example, often ask their students to read Tolstoi's *The Death of Ivan Ilych,* written a century ago (1886) but still speaking to us today. The protagonist's hollow and tormented life ends with an epiphany and his gasp of relief, "It is finished." All of his life is encapsulated in that moment that brings both meaning and cessation.

In our own times we have seen many dramatized deaths on the movie and television screens. The camera is in love with these scenes. It wants to show us the expression on face of the bad guy's face when he is riddled with bullets, or the victim who tries to say the name of the killer but just can't . . . get . . . the . . . words . . . out . . . before the moment of death. We also have a heritage of "last words" that are a mixture of the authentic, dubious, and fictitious. These utterances are often regarded as having a special epistemological status or rhetorical power precisely because of the circumstances in which they were supposed to have been made (Kastenbaum, 1993). Literary and cinematic endings and real or invented last words are examples of what might be called the social construction of the moment of death. These constructions, however, do not prove that there is invariably a decisive moment of death; they simply attest to the dramatic intensification that is achieved by focusing on one highly charged moment in time.

IT'S NOT THAT SIMPLE– FUZZING INTO THE NEXT MILLENNIUM

Today there are many who would hesitate to accept the moment of death as an unimpeachable reality. Concepts such as "clinical death" and "brain death" have become familiar to the general public as well as allied health professionals. We are aware of controversy regarding "cortical death" vs. "whole brain death" as criteria for determining the end of life. We are aware that questions regarding the criteria for determining death have escaped from the sphere of philosophy to the court room and the hospital ethics committee. We are aware of paranormal death reports that some people interpret as having experienced "temporary death," if this oxymoron be allowed. And we are aware that advocates of cryonic suspension believe that some people certified as dead might be resuscitated in the future. The destabilization of the concepts of "death" and "dead" makes it more difficult to assume that there is an actual identifiable moment of passage.

The ambiguities that have invaded our conceptions of death can be attributed in large part to technological innovations that have blurred boundaries and opened new possibilities regarding life (e.g., cloning) as well as death. From an even broader perspective, however, the life-death ambiguity is but part of a more general drift of thought away from Aristotelian logic and dichotomous categorization. The approach to interpretation and theory construction known as fuzzy logic includes some new elements, but can also be regarded as the legitimization of a previously marginalized tradition (McNeill & Freiberger, 1993). A heady example from the fairly recent past was the physicist's view that matter in motion consists neither of particles nor waves, but what might be called "wavicles." This view, in turn, has given way to even more daunting ideas about the nature of the universe. Common to most theories of the micro- or megacosmos is the principle that the observer's perspective and actions of observation must be considered as integral to our construction of the phenomena themselves.

The moment of death is an idea that flourished when the dominant mode of systematic thought was categorical, dichotomous, and absolutist: things have to be this way or that way. "It's not that simple," is the thriving contemporary view. *The observer effect* has become too well acknowledged in too many scientific disciplines for us to dismiss. In its weaker form, this proposition holds that the act of observation is itself relative to the observer's position. In the social and behavioral sciences this would certainly include not only our sensory apparatus, but also our expectations, values, previous experiences, and immediate need states. We cannot thoroughly disentangle our own being from the final moment that we have observed (or think we have observed). In its stronger form, this proposition holds that we co-create the phenomenon itself. Our own interaction with the other person and our own construction of the event influences the nature and timing of "the final moment." We recognize this influence when one person at the bedside whispers, "She is gone," while another continues to speak to the person in the bed as though she were still alive. We also recognize the observer effect when medical, religious, and interpersonal constructions of "alive" and "dead" come into conflict. But do we recognize an observer effect in the construction of the moment of death in the hospice tradition? Is hospice guided by a particular construction of the moment of death? Does hospice care contribute to creating a particular kind of final moment? We will return to these questions after other questions have been identified and more of the background has been sketched.

OBSERVING AND INTERPRETING THE LAST MOMENT

What do we know about the relationship between the perspective of the observer and the experiencer? I have seen people at what appeared to be their last moment of life. My observations were similar to what others have reported: a subtle but profound change seems to have occurred in an instant. A stillness, a repose has settled upon the person's features. The laboring person had been replaced by a statue that could have been a thousand years old or a thousand miles away.

I found myself assuming without question that the person died at the moment I noticed the transition. Upon reflection, though, I must admit that this is an inference, not an established fact. At that moment the person died to me. But did the person at the same moment also die to himself or herself? Can we even speak of the "same" moment in this situation? Altered states of consciousness are often characterized by liberation from our everyday frames of temporal experience. Furthermore, it would be careless of me to assume that other people would have observed this person's state of being in the same way. People differ in their observations and interpretations throughout the entire process of terminal illness, from early symptomatology to the moment of death and even beyond. A person may be dead to me but not to you, or vice versa. Interpretations are likely to differ more widely than observations. One might conclude, for example, that a spirit, soul, or vital essence has departed, while another holds that a non-reversible failure of life-sustaining processes has occurred, and only that.

The problem is not just that we might differ in our observations and interpretations of the moment of death. We are also inclined to attribute our own feelings, values and expectations to others, especially when their behavior is ambiguous or non-responsive. Many studies in social psychology and related disciplines have found that we often do make attributions to others that are based on our own state of mind. For example, a face in a photograph may be interpreted as friendly or hostile, heroic or criminal, depending on the expectations we have before actually seeing the photo. Psychiatrists and clinical psychologists have long been aware of the temptation to generate personal attributions to their clients (countertransference), just as the clients may be relating to the therapists as though they were significant people they had already known in their own lives (transference).

We would be naive, then, to suppose that caregivers for the terminally ill would be immune to the temptation to see something of what they hope or fear to see. The underlying reason for this possible confusion of self-and-other is simply that hospice caregivers are human, and humans often do that sort of thing. There are two other reasons, though, that are more specific to the situation. It is stating the obvious to note that dying people often grow fatigued and experience an impairment of function in many spheres, including the communicative. The less the dying person can say or do, the more that person's state of experience is open for interpretation and speculation. The other reason pertains to the core of the palliative care credo: *compassion*.

Most of the people who have made hospice what it is have the ability not only to *feel for* but also *to feel with* dying people and their families. The professional-patient distancing that became part of the medical model in the past century is replaced by a more personal and even intimate set of interpersonal exchanges. The benefits of this approach are huge, if not easily subject to measurement. However, there is also an inherent danger. At the extreme, we may be treating ourselves instead of the other person. It is our suffering, sorrow, and fear we are trying to allay. Fortunately, this extreme seems to be rare in hospice practice. Hospice philosophy and training emphasize the need to take our cues from the patients and their families, rather than to impose a predetermined set of values and procedures. Despite this valuable safeguard, however, it is probable that we do at times mix our feelings and values with those of the dying person. Accordingly, when we think of a concept as broad as "the good death" or as narrow as "the moment of death" we may be dealing with a construction that has much of our own priorities intertwined with those of patients and families. Furthermore, there are usually changes over time, some of them quite subtle, in the dying person's experiences and needs. If we are somehow locked into our own conception of the situation and do not realize this fact, then we may become increasingly out of phase with the patient's situation.

How, how much, and how often do hospice caregivers misconceive what is happening because we are not aware of our own interpretive biases and processes? These questions cannot be answered here: they require systematic research that has not yet come to light.

ON THE REALITY OF A MOMENT OF DEATH

The moment of death has been a symbolic reality for many years in many cultures. Often it is difficult to tell whether the prevailing cultural belief was literal, symbolic, or both. In medieval Europe, for example, the deathbed scene was imagined as a cosmic drama. The expulsion of the final breath marked the beginning of either salvation or damnation (Aries, 1981). The surviving artifacts suggests a mix of symbolic and literal elements. The *Ars moriendi* tracts I have had the opportunity to view bear a striking resemblance to twentieth century comic books, dominated by large, dramatic cartoon-like drawings. Readers could choose to believe in the literal reality of visible angels and demons cavorting at bedside, or interpret these as representations of good and evil, a reminder of the divine judgement to be imposed on all. The last moment with its last breath, however, provided an authenticating physicality. When the reader witnessed an actual death, there would be a strong inclination also to witness a final moment in which the same forces were present, if not visible to the eyes.

The Buddhist conception, as described by the Dalai Lama (Gyatso, 1985), offers a more complex and detailed construction of the moment of death. In keeping with Buddhist philosophy, the emphasis is on process. Dying, in a sense, happens throughout life; past, present, and future are ways of looking at an unbroken flow. Nevertheless, there are two identifiable final moments. The first marks the transition from one's life as a person among other persons. Like the medieval Christian (and many others), the Buddhist takes the cessation of breathing as evidence that death has occurred. It is at this time that the person also loses awareness of his or her own identity and habitual concerns. The person is now dead to the world, but may still be capable of new experiences. There are four "pure visionary stages," culminating in "the clear light of death." The Buddhist conception focuses consistently on the dying/dead person's phenomenological state. This eliminates or at least reduces the problem of confusing the observer's perspective with the individual's. It also proposes an after-state: something significant is still going on with the person after he or she has died, according to conventional standards.

The first of the Buddhist moments of death seems "real" in the usual sense of the term. It does not require special observations or speculations. The second ("clear light") moment of death is not observable to the living. It is "real," "symbolic," or "imaginary" depending not upon observation, then, but upon one's belief system.

But what of the simple yet compelling commonality between these two views–that the moment of death is identical with the final breath? This was the most common criterion for much of human history, and usually served well. It is also a fallible criterion, though, as at least some physicians have recognized for more than a century (Shrock,

1835). Many a person has, in fact, survived since drawing their "last breath." The advent of life support systems has further destabilized the simple idea of the last breath as marker of the moment of death. If respiration (along with other vital functions) can be supported for prolonged periods of time, then the last breath/last moment becomes a matter of medical, economic, legal, ethical, and emotional scrimmaging rather than a definitive sign.

Practical experience suggests that some people do seem to experience an identifiable moment of death that leaves us in little doubt. The last moment is not always that clear, however, and a great many people's lives come to an end without anybody being in a position to know precisely when and how. It would be overreaching to insist that there is always a clear, identifiable moment of death, but reasonable to acknowledge such endings when they do occur. (Again, there are no dependable data on frequency or circumstances.) It is an exceptional experience to bear witness to that fleeting instant in which life gives way to death, and one that deserves to be reflected upon.

WHY HAVE WE LEARNED SO LITTLE?

The introduction of hospice care focused renewed attention on dying people, especially within their interpersonal and situational contexts. The history of dying and its representation in art and culture has often featured accounts of deathbed scenes and the moment of death. We might therefore have expected that hospice philosophy and practice would lead to a major reconsideration of the deathbed scene and the moment of death. Despite the heartening growth of hospice programs around the world, however, there has been relatively little public discussion of the final scene and moment. Even the increased visibility of approaches described as "spiritual" has not materially changed the picture. Many presentations and publications now offer spiritual perspectives on terminal care, but few focus on the deathbed scene and moment of death that were so salient in the past (Kastenbaum, 1992; Kastenbaum, 1993).

This is not a critique, but rather a puzzlement. The palliative care movement has many challenges to cope with, not the least of which are management, funding, and community/professional education. Obviously, hospice organizations have to meet these challenges successfully if they are to provide end-of-life comfort to patients and families. A functionalistic and utilitarian orientation might well be expected of organizations that must continually struggle for their existence within the turmoil of current health care systems. It is perhaps surprising, however, that the deathbed scene and last moment of life, for so long the focus of spiritual concern, have become marginalized in the mainstream hospice literature. Hospice staff and volunteers are usually drawn from people with a strong sense of religious faith (Schneider & Kastenbaum, 1993). Many hospice caregivers do in fact serve by the bedside and some are present as a life ends. Isn't it a little strange, then, that there has been such a disconnect, that hospice has said so little when cultural tradition says so much about the last moments of a life?

We can only speculate about the factors that have contributed to the near-eclipse of the deathbed scene and last moment within a movement that has done so much to bring the dying person and the community together again. Other cultural traditions–even many languages and dialects–have been lost to social and technological change in recent generations. Major events, artistic creations, dominating personalities, and social movements that once were thought to be common intellectual property seem to have slipped from collective memory. Instructors at all educational levels labor to help their students make connections because so little knowledge of the past has crossed from one generation to the next. Perhaps, then, all that made the last moment of life appear to be such a spiritual crucible has simply dropped from view–leaving in its place only the cinematic death scene as a plot device.

Another possibility is that the intensely subjective character of the moment of death has no place in the objectivistic frame of discourse with which hospice and all other human service organizations must function. Quantifiable measures usually are required in the evaluation of human services. Hospice care is no exception. For example, in the large scale National Hospice Demonstration Study (Mor, Greer, & Kastenbaum, 1988), much effort was devoted to the development of reliable quantitative measures. We were quite aware of the reality and significance of subjective experience, but also equally aware that decisions about the future of the hospice movement in the United States would be made on the basis of quantifiable findings. Not surprisingly, we experienced particular difficulty with the same problem that has taxed previous and subsequent researchers: the assessment of pain.

Experts can define and operationalize the assessment of pain but, when all is said and done, only the suffering person knows, and that person often finds it very difficult to communicate his or her experience precisely and completely. How much more difficult it would have been to describe the final scene and moments of a person's life! And how little attention such descriptions would have received from number-crunching decision-makers! Perhaps, then, personal experience just does not fit into the health care regulatory system and the biomedical research enterprise: spirituality and phenomenology don't compute.

Three other possible factors might also be considered. *Source credibility* is known to have a powerful effect on our willingness to believe or even to pay attention to information. Messages from people who are considered to be relatively low in social status are often ignored by people who consider themselves superior. The feminist movement has abundant ammunition for its claim that women typically have been treated as though inferior to men, particularly in the workplace. It is also clear that most of the health care providers and volunteers who are actually there with dying people and their families are women. Furthermore, these female service providers seldom have high level professional pedestals from which to speak and write. It is possible, then, that the people who observe end-of-life experiences most closely and frequently do not have much opportunity to influence theory and practice. Their stories, well told and well heard, might enhance our understanding of the deathbed scene today: but first, we would have to think it important to know how hospice care does or does not influence the final moments of life.

Opportunities for systematic inquiry also have a significant influence on knowledge about end-of-life experiences and phenomena. Palliative care programs offer an unmatched potential for this kind of learning. Individual caregivers do learn in their own ways and are sometimes able to transmit this knowledge to others through leadership and example. What can be learned through personal experience with dying people and their families is invaluable. Personal experiences have provided the foundation for basic concepts and principles throughout the social and behavioral sciences and human service professions. Nevertheless, we also need systematic inquiry in palliative care as in other domains. As caregivers we are very much part of what happens for a limited number of people in particular circumstances.

As researchers we have the challenge of trying to identify, document and understand, applying methods and criteria that provide a different perspective on what happens.

There is an ever-increasing catalog of hospice-based research, including many contributions that have appeared in this *Journal*. Relatively few studies, however, have focused on the dynamics of the deathbed scene and/or final moment, however. In fact, most studies are somewhat remote from the crucial human experiences that appear to be at the core of the hospice mission. Thousands and thousands of people receive care through hospice programs in the last phase of their lives, but we have little opportunity to learn from their experiences in a systematic manner. Why? There are ethical, practical, and attitudinal reasons. The ethical position is clear: no palliative care (or other human service) program should compromise the welfare of its clients by intrusive research procedures. Certain types of research may therefore be rejected on ethical grounds. The practical position is also clear: hospice resources are often stretched to the maximum, and the logistics of conducting meaningful research can be very difficult. A hospice may therefore close its doors to many research efforts because they would appear to provide additional burden and stress to the organization, even if the studies themselves are not objectionable. These ethical and practical restraints on hospice-based research obviously command respect.

The attitudinal facet complicates the situation, however. Has a wall of resistance been constructed around palliative care programs based on fear and misunderstandings? Do some hospice decision-makers think of research as an alien activity rather than an inherent part of their service? Does "research" conjure the image of heartless and clueless outsiders performing strange and intrusive actions? Is there, in fact, a turf issue here, coupled with limited awareness of the ways in which mature and compassionate people can carry out meaningful research in real life (and real death) situations? Does the mere mention of "research" lead to the closing of minds and doors? Attitudinal factors are especially salient when the proposed study involves learning about the direct experiences and interactions of patients and families. Four decades ago, one of the first people to study the experiences of dying patients was repeatedly turned away by hospital administrators who, anxious themselves, could not believe that life-threatened people would actually want to share their thoughts and feelings. Herman Feifel's (1959) persistence led to the finding that many people were grateful for the opportunity to talk about their situation, and led also to the growth of the death awareness movement. Hospice staff certainly appreciate the value of communication, but may yet be leery of cooperating with research projects. There is a natural solution: the development of state-of-the-art research projects within hospice organizations. Perhaps that will be one of the achievements to note when *The Hospice Journal* performs its next twenty-year review.

Reluctance to know is a third possibility to consider. Do we really want to know how lives end? What if the findings undermine our hopes and call our beliefs into question? Perhaps we need some protective illusions if we are to continue going about our work. There does not appear to be research specific to this topic, but it has been found that even people with substantial experience as health care providers come up with personal imagined deathbed scenes that are far more romantic and idealized than the deaths they have actually been in a position to learn about (Kastenbaum & Normand, 1990). They could not help themselves from converting "expected" into "desired" death. Perhaps, just perhaps, the hospice community includes people who feel they must compartmentalize their actual experiences with deathbed scenes and final moments from their strongly-held and sustaining values. To what extent there may be a reluctance to know is one more question that awaits study.

WHAT DIFFERENCE IS HOSPICE MAKING?

Up to this point we have been raising questions about the hospice approach to understanding the deathbed scene and, more specifically, the final moment of life. We have offered the proposition that, for various reasons, hospice has not made the contribution in this sphere that might have been expected, given its philosophy, its staffing by people of faith, and the long history of religious attention to the end-of-life drama.

Now it is time to consider, if briefly, the differences that hospice seems to be making despite the limitations already noted.

Yes, Hospice Is Making a Difference

There is reason to believe that the hospice movement is accomplishing much of what it originally hoped to do, although leaders such as

Dame Cicely Saunders continually emphasize all that might yet be accomplished. Each of the following dimensions of change are likely to have a significant influence on the final scene of life for a number of people–not necessarily by their direct effect on the last moment, but by their comforting and supportive effect throughout the entire course of hospice care.

1. *Reduction of pain and pain apprehension.* Advances in pain management have enabled many terminally ill people to maintain their interpersonal relationships and both to reflect on their lives and deal with the current situation.
2. *Reduction of cognitive clouding and confusion.* Improved symptom management also has enabled more people to remain alert and responsive longer. The harsh trade-off between pain and loss of alertness has more often been avoided through procedures devised or refined by palliative care providers.
3. *Improved communication.* Less pain and less apprehension about pain, along with the protection of cognitive functioning, helps people to communicate about everything that concerns them, and also heartens others to communicate with them.
4. *Less sense of social isolation.* In turn, the maintenance of communication protects against the sense of social isolation that was so frequently noted as hospice started its mission (e.g., Glaser & Strauss, 1965; Pattison, 1977). As the last moments of life approach, the person is more likely to remain in contact with those who are most important.
5. *Family bonds preserved, not weakened.* All of the above not only benefits the dying person, but also serves to preserve or even strengthen emotional bonds within the family. Bereavement and grief have too often resulted in families splitting apart emotionally if not physically. The hospice approach of involving family members as well as directly serving the dying person contributes to family survival (Rosen, 1998).
6. *Depression may be moderated and despair prevented.* All the processes identified above have the potential for supporting a safe passage through the last phase of life. Depression and even despair remain possibilities, as will be further discussed below, but there is little doubt that many dying people–and their families–have been helped to avoid the depths of despair.

Additionally, there are at least two other ways in which hospice has been contributing indirectly to the quality of individual and family experience during the deathbed scene and final moments.

7. *Advocating a flexible approach to terminal care that is responsive to the particular people and situation.* The rule is not to have too many rules. When palliative care programs are able to follow their own philosophy successfully, they are also increasing the chances for people to experience what Avery D. Weisman (1974) has described as an "appropriate death," namely, the death one would have chosen for one's self.

8. *Helping reduce the barriers to talking about dying and death.* Public and professional education continues to be a priority for palliative care programs, as well as for those who have come to be known as "death educators." Every sensitized health care professional and family member has made it that much easier to re-integrate the deathbed scene into the communal life.

WHAT HOSPICE HAS YET TO ACCOMPLISH

It may be unrealistic and unfair to expect hospice programs to resolve problems that are deeply rooted in society or, to reverse the metaphor, problems that have been intensified by the uprooting of established belief systems and lifestyles. Nevertheless, one can at least identify some of the issues that have not been adequately addressed up to this point in time. These issues are embedded in our society's death system, the network of beliefs and practices within which how we live and how we die are intimately connected (Kastenbaum, 1998). The death system perspective does not neglect the uniqueness of an individual's experience, but, rather, attempts to discover how these experiences influence and are influenced by larger social forces.

What most concerns us here is the way in which the very end of a life is constructed today by the dying person, the family, and the health care professionals. It seems to me that for some time now our society has been losing and/or rejecting the core beliefs that have given meaning to the deathbed scene and the final moment. Emphasis must be placed on such terms as "beliefs" and "constructions." How people have actually died in the past did have some relationship to the dominant beliefs of their time, but the beliefs were not necessarily confined to nor informed by the facts. History reveals some rather hideous distortions of the deathbed experience in the rantings of "true believers" (e.g., Warton, 1826). Vested interests in all times and societies have attempted to own the deathbed scene, frequently leading to symbolic constructions that bear little resemblance to what was actually experienced. It is not necessarily the case, then, that successive generations should be obliged to maintain beliefs about the end of life that prevailed in the past. Indeed, emergent realities (such as industrialization, medical advances, and global communication) may so alter lifestyles that ideas about received ideas about dying and death cannot be expected to escape modification.

As individuals we may think we know a great deal about the state of mind–or soul–of a person approaching the transition from life to death. Many of those who read publications such as *The Hospice Journal* have personal experiences to draw upon. It would be unfortunate, though, if we substituted our personal experiences, as moving and illuminating as they might be, for the more encompassing and consensually validated knowledge that might provide us with a more reliable understanding.

Respecting the limits of our collective knowledge, then, we might simply present a series of related questions that await answer–and, if not by hospice, then by whom? Will the next dying person whose life we enter experience the final phase of life as–

- Liberation from the bonds of oppression?
- Relief from unbearable suffering?
- Entrance into a Hell of punishment for a sinful life?
- Entrance into a Heaven of inconceivable splendor?
- The supreme crucible–the occasion for a devoutly desired miracle of salvation transformation OR the verdict of damnation?
- Reunion with loved ones?
- Passing into mystery, the Great Unknown or Unknowable?
- Just crossing one more threshold in a journey of many lifetimes?
- Completing the last chapter in one's book of life?
- Junking the obsolescent, used-up and useless body?

No two of these statements are alike, even though they might appear so at first reading. Each encapsulates a different experiential construction of what it means to live, to have lived, and then to die. A person might move from one of these orientations to another during the terminal process (though not necessarily in any fixed sequence), or combine several at the same time. For example, a person might at first attempt to understand the final phase of his or her life in terms of a model that had been taken aboard in childhood. As the terminal course proceeds, however, this model may not seem to be appropriate or effective, and so the search may be on for another view of life at the edge of death.

Who knows how and why a particular person faces death with a particular set of beliefs, symbols, and meanings? Who knows how and why a particular person's terminal ordeal is alleviated, intensified, or transformed by the frame of understanding they have chosen, or which has chosen them? As companions, caregivers, and witnesses we may have some useful inferences based on the situations we have known, but as a knowledge-based field of human service, I would submit that we still know very little. Still less do we know what new ways of meeting death might be developing in our fast-changing times. For example, how will dying and death be constructed by a generation nurtured on computer games, the Internet, and virtual reality?

The ideas and passions that accompany a person to the end of life can be immensely consequential. One case history, very briefly recounted, will have to serve as our example here (Kastenbaum, 1995-1996). William McDougall, physician, psychologist, and political thinker, was among the most distinguished intellects of the 1920s and '30s. Diagnosed with terminal cancer in the prime of his life, he kept a journal in which he recorded both his daily struggles with the illness and a life review. McDougall was in terrible pain all this time, but limited his use of morphine in order to preserve his ability to think and write.

Switch our frame of reference now to current concepts and practice. The standard mental health model is the one most frequently applied to the dying person. In the past, one hoped to die in grace or, at least, not in disgrace. Today, caregivers are expected to guide terminally ill people to achieve a mentally healthful exit. The standard operating procedure includes encouraging "talking about it," reviewing and mending significant relationships, and "accepting" both one's self and death. If this model resonates with the model that has been selected by the dying person, then all may be very well. But all may not be very well if we do not recognize that we are in the grip of a particular model and in some danger of imposing it on others.

McDougall, for example, was a stalwart intellectual with a passion for thought and discovery. Was he often too intellectual in situations where emotion and human feeling would have been more appropriate? Probably so. Did he approach his own death not only with a clinical detachment, but also with a geopolitical orientation that could seem far removed from his personal ordeal? Again, probably so. Did his whole view of dying and death seem to cry out for mental health intervention? Yes, it certainly fit the profile. Would we have done the right thing to rush to McDougall to "help" him end his life in accordance with our mental health model? In all likelihood, this would have been an ignorant and arrogant action on our parts, destined only to increase his misery while offering little in return. The only possible way we might have helped would be to understand and respect his own strong alternative view of dying and death. And the only possible way we might have done that would have been to recognize our own personal and professional views for what they are: working models that do not necessarily work for everybody.

Understanding the type of understanding that people bring with them to the edge of life is perhaps even more important today than in the past. The recently-earned freedom to discuss death has also unlocked the Pandora's Box of assisted suicide. Within some frames of mind assisted suicide shines as the only way out of anxiety and despair. Within other frames of mind, assisted suicide has little attraction. There is also a frame of mind in which ideas and impulses compete fiercely with each other, with the outcome often subject to influence by interpersonal and other situational factors. It is seldom easy to understand the meanings that people bring with them in their final phase of life. There are many obstacles, including anxieties, doubts, or fears we ourselves may be carrying about. It is not out of the question that hospice programs might impose their own institutionalized barriers either by discouraging discussion of issues that are so emotionally laden or by implicitly sponsoring a "corporate image" of dying and death that caregivers are expected to foster.

Perhaps the biggest challenge today is how to nurture, support, and affirm meaning as the moment of death (or pre-terminal lapse) approaches. The model of a used-up, failed machine is all too available in a society in which even last year's amazing home computer will be obsolete next year. The person who longs for death–and perhaps is ready to have a call placed to Dr. Kevorkian–may have come to that edge of despair through a gradual attenuation of human bonds and sustaining meanings even more than the falterings of the flesh. The palliative care provider who is observant of patient and family meanings associated with the moment of death and the deathbed scene could just make the difference between affirmation and despair.

REFERENCES

Aries, P. (1981). *The hour of our death*. New York: Alfred A. Knopf.

Feifel, H. (1959). *The meaning of death*. New York: McGraw-Hill.

Glaser, B. G., & Strauss, A. (1965). *Awareness of dying*. Chicago: Aldine.

Gyatso, Tenzin, the 14th Dalai Lama (1985). *Kindness, clarity, and insight*. Ithaca: Snow Lions Publications.

Kastenbaum, R. (1992). *The psychology of death*. Second edition. New York: Springer Publishing Company.

Kastenbaum, R. (1993a). Last words. *The Monist, An International Journal of General Philosophical Inquiry*, 76, 270-290.

Kastenbaum, R. (1993b). *Is there an ideal deathbed scene?* In I. B. Corless, B. B. Germino, & W. Pittman (Eds.), *Dying, death and bereavement* (pp. 109-122). Boston: Jones & Bartlett.

Kastenbaum, R. (1995-1996). "How far can an intellectual effort diminish pain?" William McDougall's Journal as a model for facing death. *Omega, Journal of Death and Dying*, 37, 123-164.

Kastenbaum, R. (1998). *Death, society, and human experience*. Sixth edition. Boston: Allyn & Bacon.

Kastenbaum, R., & Normand, C. (1990). Deathbed scenes as expected by the young and experienced by the old. *Death Studies*, 13, 201-218.

McNeill, E., & Freiberger, P. (1993). *Fuzzy logic*. New York: Simon & Schuster.

Mor, V., Greer, D. S., & Kastenbaum, R. (Eds.) (1988). *The hospice experiment*. Baltimore: The Johns Hopkins University Press.

Pattison, E. M. (1977). *The experience of dying*. Englewood Cliffs, NJ: Prentice-Hall.

Phipps, W. E. (1988). The origin of hospices/hospitals. *Death Studies*, 12, 91-100.

Rosen, E. J. (1998). *Families facing death*. Revised edition. San Franciso: Jossey-Bass.

Saunders, C., & Kastenbaum, R. (Eds.) (1997). *Hospice care on the international scene*. New York: Springer Publishing Company.

Schneider, S., & Kastenbaum, R. (1993). Patterns and meanings of prayer in hospice caregivers: An exploratory study. *Death Studies*, 17, 471-485.

Shrock, N. M. (1835). On the signs that distinguish real from apparent death. *Transylvanian Journal of Medicine*, 13, 210-220.

Stoddard, S. (1978). *Hospice movement–a better way of caring for the dying*. New York: Stein & Day.

Tolstoi, L. (1960). *The death of Ivan Ilych*. New York: The New American Library. (Original work: 1886).

Tuchman, B. W. (1978). *A distant mirror*. New York: Alfred A. Knopf.

Warton, J. (1826). *Death-bed scenes*. (3 volumes). London: John Murray, Albemarle Street

Weisman, A. D. (1974). *The realization of death*. New York: Jason Aronson.

Index

Acquired immune deficiency syndrome
(AIDS), 15,26-27, 239-240
Advanced directives, advanced
directives and, *See*
End-of-life care
AIDS, *See* Acquired immune
deficiency syndrome (AIDS)
AIDS Resource Committee, 26
AMA, *See* American Medical
Association (AMA)
American Academy of Hospice and
Palliative Medicine, 134
American Academy of Nurses, 118
American Association of Colleges of
Nurses, 117-118
American Geriatric Society, 180
American Hospice Foundation, 187
American Hospital Association, 21
American Medical Association
(AMA), 21,114,180,228
American Nurses Association (ANA),
117-118
American Nurses Association Hall of
Fame, 12
American Pain Society, 158
American Society of Clinical
Oncology, 230
ANA, *See* American Nurses
Association (ANA)
Annenberg Center for Health
Sciences, 126
Assisted suicide, 29

Bay Area Hospice Association, 221
Bayh, Birch, 20
Bell, Bernia, 22
Bell, Howard, 25
Bereavement care, 3,5,70,187,232
Beresford, Larry, 15

Beth Israel Medical Center, 160
hospice and palliative care
advantages of, 164-165
clinical level changes and, 163
configuration of, 160-162
development management and,
165-166
hospice staff, challenges to,
162-163
palliative care professionals
challenges and, 163-164
personnel differences and, 161-162
regulatory differences and, 163
Block, Susan, 208
Blue Cross/Blue Shield Association, 21
Bonica, John, 158
Boulder County Hospice, Colorado, 22
Brenner, Paul R., 155
Brown, Robert, 18
Burt, Robert, 208
Butler, Robert, 19,208

Califano, Joseph, 19
California State Hospice Association,
221-222
Cameron, Jacqueline R., 33
Cancer pain relief, 16
CDC, *See* Centers for Disease Control
and Prevention
Center to Improve the Care of the
Dying, 113,159-200
Centers for Disease Control and
Prevention (CDC), 194
death data analysis and, 194-195
Chandler, Emily, 63
Chronic and terminal pain
control myths and, 5-6
Clarke Institute of Psychiatry, Toronto,
232
Cleeland, Charles, 159

Cleveland Clinic, 200
Collier, Earl "Duke," 21
Colorado Hospice Organization, 187
Congressional Budget Office, 21
Connecticut Hospice, 11,16,24,124,
        157,218
    physician-assisted living and,
        132-133
Connecticut State Prison System
    terminally ill prisoners and, 13
Connor, Stephen R., 15,193
Corless, Inge B., 9

Dahlin, Constance M., 75
Daniels, Kaye, 219
Davie, Karen, 31
Death, moment of, 254-255
    concepts of, 255-256
    cultures and, 258-260
    determining, criteria for, 255
    hospice movement dynamics and,
        262-264
    observing and interpreting and,
        256-258
    research and, 263-264
Death and dying, 1,3,75,88,112-113,
        131
    cultural and social challenges of,
        134,209-210,258-260
    experience of, 208
    health professionals training and, 210
    hospice care and
        changing attitudes about, 178
        costs of, 178,210
    legal and moral issues of, 134
    pain and, 210-211
    psychological, emotional and
        existential suffering and, 210
    societal perspective of, 76-77
    See also Dying patients, medical
        care of; Hospice care
Dementia, 145-146
Department of Health and Human
        Services, 223
DNR, *See* Do Not Resuscitate (DNR)
    orders and

Do Not Resuscitate (DNR) orders
        and, 110
Dobihal,Rev. Edward, 10
Dole, Robert, 19,21
Drug abuse, 207
Drug studies, 3-4
    diamorphine (heroin) and, 3-4
    morphine and, 3-5
Dying patients, medical care of
    dignity and respect of, 174
    needs and expectations of, 173
    pain management and, 170
    quality of care and, 168-169,174
        patient voice and, 171-172,
            172*fig.*,173
    satisfaction measures and, 169-171
    See also Death and dying

Edmonton Symptom Assessment
        Scale (ESAS), 186
Education for Physicians in End-of-
        Life Care (EPEC), 114
Elements of grief, 65
Eliot, T.S., 217,228
Ella Lyman Cabot Trust, 4
End-of-life
    assisted suicide and, 269
    initiatives and, 228
End-of-life care, 9,13,15,25,27
    advanced directives and, 91-94
        anticipatory care planning and,
            99-101
        current care framework and,
            95-101
    aggressive comfort treatments and,
        115-116
    case study in, 86-87
    chronically ill children and, 211
    clinical training, concepts of,
        102-105,131-132
    common shortcoming of, 111
    conclusion and, 105
    cost effectiveness and efficacy of,
        211
    cultural and social issues of, 134-135
    determining death, criteria for, 255

disease progression and, 90
Do Not Resuscitate (DNR) orders
    and, 110
emerging models and, 199,201-203
emotional and spiritual suffering
    and, 211
family caregivers and, 91
health care system and, 10,109-110,
    180
hospice services
    availability of, 211
    restrictions on admittance and,
    211
interdisciplinary approach and,
    116-117
interdisciplinary educational
    initiatives and, 119-120
legal mechanisms and, 88-89
managed care practices, 211
nursing's initiatives and, 117-119
nursing's position statement on,
    118-119
pain management and, 211
patient profile and, 89-92
physician education and, 211
psychiatric aspects of, 211
quality care models, 96,211
quality-improvement and, 211
reimbursement issues and, 104,112,
    126
service-delivery systems and, 211
studies and reports, 127-130
Toolkit of Instruments to Measure
    End-of-Life Care (TIME),
    173-174
End-of-life initiatives, 29
English, David, 17
EPEC, *See* Education for Physicians in
    End-of-Life Care (EPEC)
ESAS, *See* Edmonton Symptom
    Assessment Scale (ESAS)
Euthanasia, 213

FACCT, *See* Foundation for
    Accountability (FACCT)

Federal Hospice Study, 124
Feifel, Herman, 4,264
Foley, Kathleen M., 159,208
Foster, Zelda, 9-10
Foundation for Accountability
    (FACCT), 187-188
Foundation of Thanatology, 230
Freeman, Stanley J. J., 232
Fryer, John, 230

Gaetz, Donald, 20-21,224
Geriatric care
    life, quality of, 169
    quality of, 169
    training fundamentals of, 85,102-103
Goldenberg, Ira, 10
Gradison, Bill, 21
Grief, elements of grief, 65
Gunten, Charles F. von, 33

Hackett, Thomas, 232
Hadlock, Daniel, 18
HCFA, *See* Health Care Financing
    Administration (HCFA)
Health Care Financing Administration
    (HCFA), 20,28,126,140-141,
    143,185-186
    Hospice Demonstration Program,
    223
Heart Disease, 143-144
Hemlock Society, 208,213
Henry J. Kaiser Family Fund, 17
HHHCA, *See* Hospital Home Health
    Care Agency of California
Hill, Barbara, 18
HIV, *See* Human immunodeficiency
    virus (HIV)
HIV disease, 146-147
HOPE, *See* Health Opportunity for
    People Everywhere (HOPE)
Hospice Action, 18-19
    See also National Hospice
    Organization
Hospice and palliative care
    development of, 234-235

differences of, 114-115,125-127,
    133-135
interdisciplinary approach to,
    116-117
occupational stress and, 229
Hospice and Palliative Nurse's
    Association, 134
Hospice care
    access to
        culture and, 77-78
        economic issues, geography
            and, 80
        economic issues, insurance
            reimbursements and, 79-80,
            97-98
        race and, 77
        religious diversity and, 78-79
    admission criteria
        accepted treatments and, 82
        eligibility and, 81
        patient location and, 82-83
        primary caregiver and, 81-82
        prognosis and, 80-81
    America and, 15-16,19
    American origins of, 9-10
    basic principles and, 5,23-26,210
    challenges and barriers of, 30-31
    change, suggestions and directions
        of, 98-99
    death, moment of, 265-266
    developmental issues and, 233-234,
        236
    documenting impact of, 177-181,
        189-190
        challenges and opportunities in,
            182-184
        conclusion and, 190-191
        current efforts and, 184-189
        instrument and measure
            development and, 185
    eligibility and
        LMRP patient criteria and,
            149-150
        Medicare Hospice Benefit
            requirements and, 194

mortality criteria and, 194
rapid decline, evidence of,
    150-151,151*table*,152,
    152*table*,153
emerging models and, 199-201
    care of case management
        programs, 200-201
    disease state management
        programs, 200
    Medicaring Program and, 200
    palliative care model, 199-200
emerging trends and, 195-197
end of life
    construction of, 266-270
family support and, 4,25-26
federal scrutiny and, 179,250
focus of
    changes in decision-making,
        133,211-212
    changes in financial arrangements,
        133-134,211-212
future of, 226-228
future scenarios and, 201-202,
    202*fig.*,203
home care and, 2,4,25-26
home health agency and, 224-226
impact of, 179
instrument and measure
        development and
    Edmonton Symptom Assessment
        Scale (ESAS), 186
    Hospice Quality of Life measure,
        185
    McGill Quality of Life Index,
        185-186
    Missoula-VITAS Quality of Life
        Index, 185-186
    National Hospice Work Group
        (NHWG), 186
    National Hospice Work Group
        (NHWG) and NHO task
        force, 186
    NHO Family Satisfaction
        Survey, 186
    Outcomes and Assessment
        Information Set (OASIS), 186

Support Team Assessment System (STAS), 186
interdisciplinary approach and, 116-117
interdisciplinary educational initiatives and, 119
International origins and, 1,3
limitations of, 180-181
Medicare Hospice Benefit requirements and
emerging trends and, 195-197
mission of, 197-199,203,248, 250-251
new initiatives and, 193-195
non-cancer patients and, 30, 140-141
challenge of, 141-142
philosophy and, 5,20,22,25,98,110
professional organizations and care delivery, changes in, 134
public understanding and, 29-30, 220
spirituality and, 11,26,261 (*See also* Spiritual journeys; Spirituality, hospice movement and)
staff stress and
major stressors of, 240-242
professional conflicts and, 242
research literature, review of, 243
research of, 237-239
training programs and, 179
volunteers and, 221
See also Beth Israel Medical Center; Death and dying; End of life care
Hospice Care commemorative postage stamp, 30
Hospice Consortium for Quality Care, 187
Hospice Inc., *See* Connecticut Hospice
Hospice leadership, 219
Hospice movement
committee structure and, 23

contribution of, 114
education and, 17,23-24
evolution of, 223
health care and medical ethics and, 12
history of, 1,6
United States and, 123-125, 248-249
inception and development of, 1-4, 17,22-23,198-199,234
nursing responsibility and, 13, 110
origins of, 155-157,230-232,254
research and teaching in, 1-5
standards of care and, 23,110
See also End-of-life care; Palliative care
Hospice of Marin, 16-17,24,157
Hospice of North Iowa Center, 249-250
Hospice Quality of Life measure, 185
Hospital Home Health Care Agency of California (HHHCA), 219
Houde, Raymond, 158
House Ways & Means Committee, 21
Human immunodeficiency virus (HIV), 146-147

Institute of Medicine (IOM), 119,169, 184,228
Institute of Medicine's End-of-Life Committee, 113
International Council of Nurses, 118
International hospice movement, 1
International Work Group on Death, Dying and Bereavement, 11, 231
IOM, *See* Institute of Medicine (IOM)

JCAHO, *See* Joint Commission on Accreditation of Healthcare Organizations (JCAHO)
Joint Commission on Accreditation of Healthcare Organizations (JCAHO), 29,183,186,223

Joint Commission on Accreditation of
     Hospitals, 24,125

Kastenbaum, Robert, 253
Kennedy, Edward, 19
Krammer, Lisa M., 33
Kubler-Ross, Elizabeth, 4,10,156,
     207-208,220,230
Kutscher, Austin, 230

Lamers, William Jr., 17
Lifton, Robert Jay, 231
Lindemann, Erich, 232
Liver disease, 147-148
LMRP, *See* Local Medical Review
     Policy (LMRP)
Local Medical Review Policy (LMRP),
     143-144,147,149
Lyall, Alan, 233,237
Lynn, Joanne, 200

MacGregor, Ann, 247
Magno, Josefina, 19,22
Mahoney, John J., 22,28
Massachusetts General Hospital, 232
McDougall, William, 268-269
McGill Quality of Life Index, 185-186
McKell, Douglas, 18
MDP, *See* Missoula Demonstration
     Project (MDP)
Medicaid hospice benefit, 27
Medical expenses, 212-213
Medicare Fiscal Intermediaries, 143,
     153
Medicare hospice benefit, 15,223,227
     eligibility, reimbursement effects
          and, 140-141
     eligibility criteria and, 81,83-84,97,
          124,140,194
     enactment of, 19-21,27
     end-of-life care, impact of, 202
     future scenarios and, 201-203
     limitations of, 202
Merriman, Melanie P., 177

Minority and Non-Cancer access Task
     Forces, 27
Missoula Demonstration Project
     (MDP), 114,190
Missoula-VITAS Quality of Life
     Index, 185-186
Morfogen, Zachary, 17-18,222
Morphine, 3,5-6
     home care and, 6
     See also Drug studies; Pain and
          symptom control
Mount, Balfour, 5,11,218,231,233
Mount Holyoke College, 11
Muir, J. Cameron, 33

National Hospice Demonstration
     Study, 261
National Hospice Education Project
     (NHEP), 20-21
National Hospice Organization (NHO),
     15-19,126,140-141,186,188,
     190,193
     assisted suicide, opposition to, 29
     development and role of, 27-30,237
     history of, 9,15,17-24
     major functions of, 31
     non-cancer disease, guidelines for,
          142-143
          dementia and, 145-146
          heart disease and, 143-144
          HIV disease and, 146-147
          liver disease and, 147-148
          pulmonary disease and, 144-145
          renal disease and, 148
          stroke and coma, 148-149
     pain management, study of, 179
     Standards and Accreditation
          Committee, 222-223
     study of
          cost effectiveness of hospice
               care, 179-180
National Hospice Study (NHS), 185,
     190,238
National Hospice Week, 24
National Hospice Work Group
     (NHWG), 186

National Hospice Work Group
(NHWG) and NHO task
force, 186
National League of Nursing, 118
Neuropathic pain, 34-36
See also Symptom control,
neuropathic pain and
New York University (NYU), 118
NHEP, *See* National Hospice
Education Project (NHEP)
NHO, *See* National Hospice
Organization (NHO)
NHO Family Satisfaction Survey, 186
NHS, *See* National Hospice Study (NHS)
NHWG, *See* National Hospice Work
Group (NHWG)
North American Conference on Caring
for Terminally Ill People
with AIDS, 26
Nursing home reimbursements, 27-29

OASIS, *See* Outcomes and Assessment
Information Set (OASIS)
O'Connor, Patrice, 123
Office of Inspector General (OIG), 28
Ohio Hospice Organization (OHO),
188-189
OHO, *See* Ohio Hospice Organization
OIG, *See* Office of Inspector General
(OIG)
Open society, 206-207
Open Society Institute's Center on
Crime, Community and
Culture, 214
Operation Restore Trust (ORT), 28,80
ORT, *See* Operation Restore Trust
(ORT)
Outcomes and Assessment Information
Set (OASIS), 186
*Oxford Textbook of Palliative
Medicine*, 2-3,157

Pain
assessment of, 262
physical elements of, 6

psychological elements of, 6
social elements of, 6
spiritual elements of, 6
Pain and symptom management
criteria and standards for, 96,198
holistic approach to, 220
physician training and, 102
regional and geographic variations
and, 96-97
study of, 179
Pain control, 1,3
Palliative care, 1,5-6,29
activities initiated and, 159-160
definition of, 111,125
development of, 135
goals of, 111-112,115-116
hospital and medical practice
resistance to, 10
origins of, 114,157-160
precepts of, 111-112,115
quality of life, dimensions of, 116
training fundamentals and, 85,
102-103,115,126
See also End-of-life care; Hospice;
Hospice care; Hospice
movement
Palliative Care Program, 158
Panetta, Leon, 20-21
Parkes, Colin Murray, 3,10
Patient Self-Determination Act, 93
Philadelphia Ars Moriendi group,
230-231
Physician assisted suicide, 132-133,
213-214
Portney, Russell, 159
Prem, Patricia, 208
Princess Margaret Hospital, 233
Project on Death in America, 113,
205-215
Alliance for Aging Research,
212-213
Faculty Scholars Program and,
211-212
Grantmakers Concerned with Care
at the End of Life, 214
Grants Program and, 211-212

mission of, 205-206
National Committee on Financing
Care at the End of Life, 212
Pulmonary disease, 144-145

Reagan, Ronald, 20
Reflections on Death in America, 205
Renal disease, 148
Rezendes, Dennis, 17-18,20,24-25,222
Robert Wood Johnson Foundation,
110-111,117-120,159,228
Robert Wood Johnson Foundation's
Last Acts, 29,111-113,119
Rogers, Alice, 158
Rogers, Joy, 237
Rothman, David, 208
Royal Victoria Hospital Palliative
Care Unit, 237

Saunders, Cicely, 1,10,16,19,114,155,
157-158,198,218,231,233-234,
239,265
Seaver, Anna Mae Halgrim, 167-168
Shedd, Charlotte, 18,23
Sherman, Deborah Witt, 109
Soros, George, 205
Southern California Hospice
Association, 221
Spillman, Ken, 230
Spiritual journeys, 64-65
caregivers and post-traumatic stress
disorder, 66-68
phases of, 64-68
sensory spirituality and, 71-72
Spirituality
hospice movement and, 63-64,
261-262
alternative therapies and, 68,70
the arts and, 68-70
integrating spirituality and the
arts, 68-70
psychosociospiritual care and,
70-72
St. Christopher's Hospice, 2-5,16,158,
218

St. Christopher's Hospice Information
Service, 5
St. Joseph's Hospice, 2,4-5
St. Luke's Hospital, London, 2-3,5
St. Luke's Hospital, New York, 124,
158,200
State Pain Initiatives in United States,
159
Stoddard, Sandal, 19
Stroke and coma, 148-149
Stuart, Brad, 139
Study to Understand Prognosis and
Preferences for Outcomes
and Risks of Treatment
(SUPPORT), 159
SUPPORT, *See* Study to Understand
Prognosis and Preferences
for Outcomes and Risks of
Treatment (SUPPORT)
SUPPORT Study, 110-111,113,117,
120,134,159-160,180-181,190
Support Team Assessment System
(STAS), 186
Sweetser, Carleton, 5
Symptom control, 1,3,33-34
for anorexia/cachexia syndrome,
47-48
etiology of, 47
pharmacological interventions
and, 47-48
for asthenia/fatigue, 48-50
anemia and, 50
etiology of, 49
pain intensity and, 49
pathophysiology of, 49
psychological components and,
50
for bowel obstruction, 45-47
nausea and vomiting and, 46-47
pharmacological management
and, 46
standard approach to, 45
for constipation, 40,40*fig.*
peristalsis stimulating laxatives
and, 41
softening laxatives and, 41

for delirium and terminal agitation, 50-52
  etiology of, 51
  Memorial Delirium Assessment Scale and, 51
  terminal delirium, differences of, 52
for depression, 52-54
  hopelessness and anhedonia, key signs of, 53
  pharmacologic therapy and, 53-54
  risk factors of, 52-53
for diarrhea, 41-42,42*table,*43
for dyspnea, 36-37
  Edmonton Symptom Assessment System and, 37
  etiology of, 37
  non-pharmacologic therapy and, 39
  oxygen therapy and, 38
  pathophysiology of, 37
  pharmacological treatment and, 37,37*fig.,*38,38*fig.,*39
  Support Team Assessment Schedule and, 37
for nausea and vomiting, 43-44, 44*fig.,*45*fig.*
  antiemetic research and, 44
  non-pharmacotherapy and, 44
  pathophysiology of, 43
  pharmacotherapy and, 43-44
for neuropathic pain, 34-36
  pharmacologic interventions and, 35-36

Tax Equity and Fiscal Responsibility Act of 1982, 21
  See also Medicare hospice benefit
Tehan, Claire B., 217
Teno, Joan M., 167,188
Terminal illness, 1,25
The Hospice Journal, 254
Thomas, Ewart V., 23-24
Thompson, Marilyn, 17

TIME, *See* Toolkit of Instruments to Measure End-of-Life Care (TIME)
Toolkit of Instruments to Measure End-of-Life Care (TIME), 173-174,188
Twycross, Robert, 3-5

UHF, *See* United Hospital Fund (UHF) Hospital Palliative Care Initiative
United Hospital Fund (UHF) Hospital Palliative Care Initiative, 161
University of Rochester Cancer Center, 218
Ursuline College, 118

Vachon, Mary L. S., 229
Vickery, Ann Morgan, 21

Wald, Florence, 4,9-13,16,124,157, 218,231
Wald, Henry, 11
Walsh, Declan, 200
Walsh, William B., 247
Warner Lambert, 21,23-24
Weisman, Avery, 232
Wessel, Morris, 10
Westbrook, Hugh, 20,224
WHO Standards for Cancer Pain Relief, 159
W.K. Kellogg Foundation, 24
Wollner, David, 85
World Health Organisation, 5
  Cancer and Palliative Care Unit, 5-6

Yale-New Haven Medical Center, 10
Yale University, 4,10,12

Zabel, William D., 208
Zorza, Victor, 18-19
Zuckerman, Connie, 85

ACADEMIC/PROFESSIONAL OVERSEAS DISTRIBUTORS, SALES REPRESENTATIVES & JOBBERS

UNITED KINGDOM

ATTENTION INTERNATIONAL DISTRIBUTORS & SALES REPS:
No more transatlantic return costs! Haworth Press books now available from the UK!
Book Representation & Distribution, Ltd
Dan Levey, Managing Director
Hadleigh Hall, London Road
Hadleigh SS7 2DE
Tel: 01702 552912
Fax: 01702 556095
E-mail: mail@bookreps.com

London
Celia Stocks
85 Church Street, Gt Burstead
CM11 2TS
Tel: 01277 657091
E-mail: CELIA@mstocks9.freeserve.co.uk

Surrey, Sussex, Hertfordshire, Bedfordshire Kent, Essex, Suffolk, Norfolk, Cambridgeshire, Lincolnshire, Buckinghamshire, Northamptonshire, Leicestershire, Nottinghamshire, Eire, Northern Ireland
Robin Wyn Jones
2, Onslow Close, Hatfield AL10 8QJ
Tel: 01707 696256
E-mail: robwynj@netscape.met

Cornwall, Devon, Dorset, Hampshire, Somerset, Avon, Wiltshire, Berkshire, Oxfordshire, Glostershire, Warwickshire, West Midlands, Hereford & Worcestershire, Glamorgans, Gwent, Dyfed, Powys
Eleanor Cripps
4, Lytes Cary Road, Keynsham
Bristol, BS18 1XD
Tel: 01179 837326
E-mail: elliecripps@blueyonder.co.uk

Gwynedd, Clwyd, Shropshire, Staffordshire, Derbyshire, Cheshire, Merseyside, Gtr. Manchester, Yorkshire, Humberside, Lancashire, Cumbria, Cleveland, Durham, Tyne & Wear, Northumberland, Scotland
Darren Denton
20 Castle Hill View
Heckmondwike, WF16 OBX
Tel: 01924 404509
E-mail: darren.denton@btopenworld.com

GERMANY, AUSTRIA & SWITZERLAND
Bernd Feldmann
Am Kanal 25
D–16515 Oranienburg, Germany
Tel: +49–3301/20 57 75
Fax: +49–3301/20 57 82
E-mail: BFeldmann@snafu.de

SCANDINAVIA
Sweden, Denmark, Norway, Finland, Iceland, Greenland
Jan Norbye
Jomsborgvej 22, DK–3650 Ølstykke
Denmark
Tel: (+45) 47174048
Fax: (+45) 47175200
E-mail: norbye@image.dk

GREECE
Katia Zevelekakis
P.O. Box 70 833
GR–166 05 Voula, Greece
(30) 210 7258397
Fax: (30) 1–899–1873 or (30) 1–725–7715
E-mail: katiaz@zevelekakis.gr

ITALY
Flavio Marcello
Marcello s.a.s.
Via Belzoni, 12, 35121 PADOVA – ITALY
Tel: [39] 049 8360671
Fax: [39] 049 8786759
E-mail: marcellosas@tuttopmi.it

SPAIN & PORTUGAL
Iberian Book Services
Peter Prout
Sector Islas, Bioque, 12 1° B
28760 Tres Cantos (Madrid) Spain
Tel: (3491) 803–49–81
Fax: (3491) 803–59–36
E-mail: pprout@jazzfree.com

RUSSIA
Mezhdunarodnaya Kniga
Bolsaya Jakimanka ul. 39.
Moscow 117049 Russia
Tel: 7 095 23384611 / Fax: 7 095 2302117

ISRAEL
Richard Sherman
Academon Import Dept.
P.O. Box 41, Jerusalem, Israel
Tel: (972) 2–588–2163
Fax: (972) 2–581–5558
E-mail: richard@academon.co.il

CENTRAL & EASTERN EUROPE
Hungary
• Dr. Laszlo Horvath
  Bem u. 5
  H-1047 Budapest, Hungary
  Tel: 36–1–379–5032 / Fax: 36–1–379–5842
  E-mail: laszloaw@mail.matav.hu
• LIBROTRADE
  Marta Dobos
  11–1173 Budapest, Pesti ut 237
  P.O. Box 1656
  Budapest, Pf 126, Hungary

Croatia
• Rado & Straus
  Book Trade & Sub. Agency
  P. Hatza 16, 10000, Zagreb, Croatia
  Tel/Fax: +385–1–48–73–414
  E-mail: rado-straus@zg.tel.hr
• TAMARIS
  Petrinjska 11, 10000
  Zagreb, Croatia
  Tel: 00385–1–48–13–356
  Fax: 00385–1–48–13–357
  E-mail: tamaris@tamaris.hr

Estonia
• Allecto, Junkentali 32-5
  EE0001 Tallinn
• AB Marefest, Ltd, Akadeemia 21G
  EE0026 Tallinn

Latvia
Aperto Libro 31, Krisjana Barona St.
LV 1763 Riga

Lithuania
Humanitas, Donelaicio 52, 3000 Kaunas

Poland
ABE Marketing
Marek Nowakowski
Ul. Grzybowski 37A, 00-855 Warsaw, Poland
Tel: 48 22 6540675 / Fax: 48 22 6520767
E-mail: mareknow@ikp.pl

Slovakia & Czech Republic
Myris Trade, Ltd.
PO Box 2, V Stihlach 1311
142 01 Prague 4, Czech Republic

Yugoslavia
Predrag Durkovic
Data Status Subscription Agency
P.O. Box 502, YU – 11000 Beograd
YUGOSLAVIA – Serbia
Tel/Fax: 381–11–361–2932
E-mail: dpredrag@datastatus.co.yu

THE MIDDLE EAST
Kuwait
The Kuwait Bookshops Co. Ltd.
• Al–Muthanna Complex
  Fahed Al–Salem Street
  P.O. Box 2942, 13030–Safat–Kuwait
  Tel: 2424266, 2424289
  Fax: 2420558
  E-mail: kbs@ncc.moc.kw
• Thunaayan AL–Ghanim Building
  Al–Sour Street
  Tel: 2434225/2435347
• Ahmadi Branch
  Souk Al–Ahmadi
  Tel: 3982590

Jordan
Jordan Book Centre Company
Gabi Sharbain
P.O. Box 301 Al Jubeiha
Amman 11941 Jordon
Tel: (962) 6–515–1882
Fax: (962) 6–515–2016
E-mail: jbc@go.com.jo

AUSTRALIA, NEW ZEALAND & PAPUA NEW GUINEA
• James Bennett Pty. Ltd.
  Marika Whitfield
  #3 Narabang Way
  Belrose, NSW 2085 Australia
  Tel: 61–2–9986–7009
  Fax: 61–2–9986–7031
  E-mail: mwhitfield@bennett.com.au
• DA Information Services Pty. Ltd.
  648 Whitehorse Road
  Mitcham, Victoria 3132 Australia
  Tel: 61–3–9210–7777
  Fax: 61–3–9210–7788
  E-mail: service@dadirect.com.au
• Barbican Book Agencies
  Contact: Owen Nicholls
  Western Australia 6008
  E-mail: onicholls@bigpond.com.au
• Auspub Agencies
  Contact: Russ Sheldrick
  Sout Australia 5097
  Ph./Fax (08) 8264 4798

- Hopwood Enterprises
  Contact: Andrew Hopwood
  Tasmania 7024
  E-mail: ahopwood@bigpond.com.au
- Book Outlet Agencies
  Contact: Brian Holden
  Queensland 4074
  Email: bookout@bigpond.com.au
- Valkyrie Book Agencies
  Contact: Margaret Allston
  New South Wales 2100
  Ph. (02) 9975 2506

AFRICA
Kenya
- Ethan Atkin
  Cranbury International
  7 Clarendon Ave., Suite 2
  Montpelier, VT 05602
  Tel: 1–802–223–6565
  Fax: 1–802–223–6824
  E-mail: eatkin@cranburyinternational.com
- Dr. Robert Obudho
  Suba Books & Periodicals
  Private Bag 51336
  ICIPE Bldg (old), Suite 14A
  Chiromo Campus
  Riverside Drive, Nairobi, Kenya
  Tel: 254–2–449231 or 449186
  Fax: 254–2–444110

Ghana
Rev. Emmanual K. Aryee
Managing Director
Methodist Book Depot
P.O. Box 100, Accra, Ghana

South Africa
(also Botswana & Namibia)
Academic Marketing
Services (Pty) Ltd
Michael Brightmore, Managing Dir.
P.O. Box 411738
Craighall 2024, South Africa
Tel: (011) 447 7441 / Fax: (011) 447 2024
E-mail: ams@icon.co.za

Uganda
Mukono Bookshop Ltd.
P.O. Box 7, Diamond Trust Building
Kampala, Uganda
Tel: 242041 or 256402

Zimbabwe
Publishers' Representative
Barbie Keene
P.O. Box MR 67, Marlborough
Harare, Zimbabwe
Tel/Fax: (263–4) 300751

ASIA & THE PACIFIC
India
- Ethan Atkin
  Cranbury International
  7 Clarendon Ave., Suite 2
  Montpelier, VT 05602
  Tel: 1–802–223–6565
  Fax: 1–802–223–6824
  E-mail: eatkin@cranburyinternational.com
- Dipak Kumar Guha
  P.O. Box 3205
  New Delhi 110013, India
  Tel/Fax: 91–11–5500998

Japan
MK International, Ltd.
Mrs. Masako Kitamura
1–50–7–203 Itabashi
Itabashi-ku, Tokyo 173, Japan
Tel: 81–3–5375–3287
Fax: 81–3–5375–3286

South Korea
Information & Culture Korea
Se-Yung Jun
473–19 Seokyo-dong, Mapo-ku
Seoul, 121–842, South Korea
Tel: 82–2–3141–4791
Fax: 82–2–3141–7733
E-mail: ickseoul@kornet.net

Pakistan
Tahir M. Lodhi
Publishers, Consultants
& Representatives
14–G, Canalberg H.S., Thoker Niaz Baig
Post Office–53700, LAHORE–PAKISTAN
Tel: +92 42 5412680
Fax: +92 42 5412690
E-mail: tml@brain.net.pk

People's Republic of
China & Hong Kong
Cassidy and Associates
Thomas V. Cassidy
375 Trailsend Drive
Torrington, CT 06790 USA
Tel: (860) 482–3030
Fax: (860) 482–0778
E-mail: chinacas@prodigy.net
- Stockholding Supplier
  Mr. Leung Wah, Director
  Park's Book Shop LTD
  Rex House, 1st Floor Flat A
  648 Nathan Road
  Mongkok, Kowloon, Hong Kong
- China: Sub-agent
  Ms. Sun Jie
  C/O CCPH
  No. 5 Jiannei Dajie
  Beijing 100732, CHINA
  Tel: 0118610–65137744
  Fax: 0118610–65273168
  E-mail: yxq@office.cass.net.cn

Philippines, Guam
& Pacific Trust Territories
I.J. Sagun Enterprises, Inc.
Tony P. Sagun, President
2 Topaz Rd., Greenheights Village
Ortigas Ave. Extension Tatay, Rizal
Republic of the Philippines
P.O. Box 4322 (Mailing Address)
CPO Manila 1099
Tel: 632–660–5479 / Fax: 632–660–8466
E-mail: apsagun@amdg.com.ph

Singapore, Taiwan, Indonesia,
Thailand & Malaysia
APAC Publishers
Steven Goh
31, Tannery Lane
#07–01 Dragon Land Building
Singapore 347788
Tel: (65) 6844–7333/6747–8662
Fax: (65) 6747–8916
E-mail: SERENA@APACMEDIA.COM.SG
- Malaysia
  Arumugam Kaliappan
  c/o APAC Publishers

LATIN AMERICA & THE CARIBBEAN
Mexico
Linda Sametz
Ave. Fuente de las Aguilas 131
Tecamachalco
53950 Mexico, Edo de Mexico
E-mail: lindas@att.net.mx
- Mexico: Sub-agent
  Sistemas Biblioinforma S.A. de C.V.
  9a. Oriente No. 8, Col. Isadro Fabela
  Deleg. Tlalpan, 14030, Mexico D.D.
  Tel: 52–56–65–38–43
  Fax: 52–56–66–20–13
  E-mail: 104552.2267@compuserve.com

Central America
Jose Rios
Apartado Postal 370-A
Ciudad Guatemala, Guatemala
Tel/Fax: (502) 443–0472
E-mail: publieduca@hotmail.com

South America
Mr. Julio Emod
Rua Joauim Tavora 629
04015-001 Sao Paulo, Brazil
Tel: (55–11) 571–1122
Fax: (55–11) 575–6876
E-mail: emod@harbra.com.br

Puerto Rico, the U.S. Virgin
Islands & the Caribbean
David A. Rivera
MSC 609 #89 Ave. De Diego
Suite 105, San Juan, PR 00927–5831
Tel: (787) 764–3532
Fax: (787) 764–4774
E-mail: drrivera@coqui.net

SALES & TRANSLATION RIGHTS
For inquiries regarding business
proposals for open sales territories or co-
representation, please contact:
Margaret Tatich
Sales & Publicity Manager
The Haworth Press, Inc.
10 Alice Street
Binghamton, NY 13904–1580
Tel: (607) 722-5857 ext. 321
Fax: (607) 722-6362
E-mail: mtatich@haworthpressinc.com

Translations
For inquiries regarding foreign rights
(primarily translations), please contact:
Anu Hanson
Foreign Rights Administrator
The Haworth Press, Inc. / ATMARR
P.O. Box 3253, Fort Lee, NJ 07024
Tel: (201) 242-5548
Fax: (201) 242-9446
E-mail: ANUH8@aol.com

CANADA: RETURNS ONLY!
The Haworth Press, Inc.
c/o Nexar Book Distributors
74 Rolark Drive
Scarborough, Ontario M1R 4G2 Canada
- No telephone calls
- Freight must be prepaid
- No correspondence
- No collect shipments

For Product Safety Concerns and Information please contact our EU
representative GPSR@taylorandfrancis.com
Taylor & Francis Verlag GmbH, Kaufingerstraße 24, 80331 München, Germany

www.ingramcontent.com/pod-product-compliance
Lightning Source LLC
Chambersburg PA
CBHW060152280326
41932CB00012B/1727